# Treating the Dental Patient with a Developmental Disorder

# Treating the Dental Patient with a Developmental Disorder

Edited by Karen A. Raposa
and Steven P. Perlman

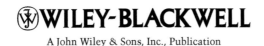

A John Wiley & Sons, Inc., Publication

This edition first published 2012 © 2012 by John Wiley & Sons, Inc

Wiley-Blackwell is an imprint of John Wiley & Sons, formed by the merger of Wiley's global Scient ific, Technical and Medical business with Blackwell Publishing.

*Editorial Offices*
2121 State Avenue, Ames, Iowa 50014-8300, USA
The Atrium, Southern Gate, Chichester, West Sussex, PO19 8SQ, UK
9600 Garsington Road, Oxford, OX4 2DQ, UK

For details of our global editorial offices, for customer services and for information about how to apply for permission to reuse the copyright material in this book please see our website at www.wiley.com/wiley-blackwell.

*Library of Congress Cataloging-in-Publication Data*
Treating the dental patient with a developmental disorder / edited by Karen A. Raposa and Steven P. Perlman.
     p. ; cm.
   Includes bibliographical references and index.
   ISBN 978-0-8138-2393-5 (pbk. : alk. paper)
   I. Raposa, Karen A.   II.  Perlman, Steven P.
   [DNLM:   1.  Dental Care for Disabled.    2.  Dentist-Patient Relations.    3.  Developmental Disabilities.    4.  Needs Assessment.    5.  Oral Hygiene.    WU 470]
   617.0087′5–dc23
                                                       2012005126
A catalogue record for this book is available from the British Library.

Wiley also publishes its books in a variety of electronic formats. Some content that appears in print may not be available in electronic books.

Set in 9.5/12pt Palatino by SPi Publisher Services, Pondicherry, India

**Disclaimer**

1   2012

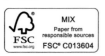

## Dedication

To my son Tommy for giving me the inspiration.
To my husband, Russ, for driving my motivation.
To my son RJ for encouraging my dedication.
And to my daughter, Brandi-Lee, for providing me with the
fortification to press on no matter what challenges I may face.
I love you all!

Karen Raposa

To my loving wife, Harriet, daughters, Meredith and Brette, and our loved
ones Michael, Jeff, and grandchildren Rachael, Eve, Alexandra, and
Matthew.

To my partner, Michael Koidin, and office staff who have been with me
forever and provided a quality dental home for thousands of families of
loved ones with special health care needs.

To my Special Olympics family, who in the second half of my career enabled
me to create a global movement and encounter countless wonderful, caring,
compassionate, and competent dental professionals, including all the
contributors to this book.

I am truly blessed to have you all in my life.

Steven Perlman

# Contents

# Contributors

## Editors

**Steven P. Perlman, DDS, MScD, DHL (Hon)**
Global Clinical Director, Special Olympics Special Smiles
Clinical Professor of Pediatric Dentistry
Henry M. Goldman School of Dental Medicine
Boston University
Boston, Massachusetts
Private pediatric dentistry practice
Lynn, Massachusetts

**Karen A. Raposa, RDH, MBA**
Speaker and author
Raynham, Massachusetts

## Consulting Editors

**Paul James Vankevich, DMD, CDR, DC, USN (RET)**
Assistant Clinical Professor
Department of General Dentistry
Tufts University School of Dental Medicine
Boston, Massachusetts

**Burton Wasserman, DDS, DABSCD**
Founder and Chair
Department of Dentistry
New York Hospital Queens
Flushing, New York

## Contributors

**Joseph M. Calabrese, DMD, FACD**
Assistant Dean of Students
Assistant Professor
Henry M. Goldman School of Dental Medicine
Boston University
Boston, Massachusetts
Director of Dental Medicine
Hebrew Senior Life
Boston, Massachusetts
Clinical Instructor
Department of Oral Health
Policy and Epidemiology
Harvard School of Dental Medicine
Boston, Massachusetts

**Debra Cinotti, DDS**
Associate Professor
Director, General Practice Residency Program

Stony Brook University Hospital, Department of Dentistry
Program Coordinator, Dental Care for Persons with Developmental Disabilities
Stony Brook University School of Dental Medicine
Stony Brook, New York

**Matthew Cooke, DDS, MD, MPH**
Assistant Professor
Department of Anesthesiology
School of Dental Medicine
University of Pittsburgh
Pittsburgh, Pennsylvania
Department of Pediatric Dentistry
School of Dentistry
Virginia Commonwealth University
Richmond, Virginia

**Ann-Marie C. DePalma, CDA, RDH, MEd, FADIA, FAADH**
Continuing Education Speaker
Stoneham, Massachusetts

**Paul S. Farsai, DMD, MPH**
Associate Professor
Director of Evidence-Based Dentistry and Behavioral Sciences
Department of General Dentistry
Henry M. Goldman School of Dental Medicine
Boston University
Boston, Massachusetts
Private Practice
Swampscott, Massachusetts

**Clive Friedman, DDS**
Diplomate American Board Pediatric Dentistry
Assistant Clinical Professor, Schulich School of Medicine and Dentistry
Western University of Ontario
London, Ontario, Canada
Assistant Clinical Professor, University of Toronto School of Dentistry

Toronto, Ontario, Canada
Private Practice Pediatric Dentistry, London, Ontario, Canada

**Cristina E. Garcia-Godoy, DDS, CCRP, MPH**
Associate Professor and Director of Clinical Research
College of Dental Medicine
Nova Southeastern University
Fort Lauderdale, Florida

**Federico Garcia-Godoy, DDS, MA**
Dean and Founder
Iberoamerican School of Graduate Dentistry
Department of Pediatric Dentistry
INCE University
Santo Domingo, Dominican Republic
Chair, Special Olympics, Dominican Republic

**Paul Glassman, DDS, MA, MBA**
Professor and Director of Community Oral Health
Director of the Pacific Center for Special Care
Arthur A. Dugoni School of Dentistry
University of the Pacific
San Francisco, California

**Matthew Holder, MD, MBA**
Executive Director
American Academy of Developmental Medicine and Dentistry
Global Medical Advisor, Special Olympics International and CEO, Underwood and Lee Clinic

**Henry Hood, DMD**
Clinical Associate Professor
Department of Orthodontics, Pediatric Dentistry & Special Care
School of Dentistry
University of Louisville
Louisville, Kentucky

Chief Clinical Officer
Underwood & Lee Clinic
Louisville, Kentucky
Co-founder, American Academy of
Developmental Medicine and Dentistry

**Martha Ann Keels, DDS, PhD**
Division Chief, Pediatric Dentistry
Duke Children's Hospital and Health
System
Durham, North Carolina

**Ray A. Lyons, DDS, FADPD, DABSCD**
Chief of Special Needs Dentistry
New Mexico Department of Health
Albuquerque, New Mexico

**Luc A.M. Marks, DDS, MSc, PhD**
Professor and Chair, Center for Special
Care in Dentistry
Dental School
Ghent University
Ghent, Belgium

**Christine E. Miller, RDH, MHS, MA**
Associate Professor and Director of
Community Programs
Founder, Pacific Special Care Clinic
University of the Pacific Arthur A. Dugoni
 School of Dentistry
San Francisco, California

**Rick Rader, MD, FAAIDD**
Director, Morton J. Kent Habilitation
Center
Orange Grove Center
Chattanooga, Tennessee

**Maureen Romer, DDS, MPA, FADPD,
DABSCD**
Associate Professor & Director, Special
Care Dentistry

Arizona School of Dentistry & Oral Health
A.T. Still University
Mesa, Arizona

**Timothy P. Shriver, PhD**
Chairman, Board of Directors, and Chief
Executive Officer
Special Olympics

**Jo Ann Simons, MSW**
President/CEO
Cardinal Cushing Centers
Hanover, Massachusetts
Disability Advisor
Ruderman Family Foundation
United States and Israel

**David Albert Tesini, DMD, MS, FDS
RCSEd**
Associate Clinical Professor
Department of Pediatric Dentistry
Tufts University School of Dental
Medicine
Boston, Massachusetts

**H. Barry Waldman, DDS, MPH, PhD**
Distinguished Teaching Professor
Department of General Dentistry
School of Dental Medicine
Stony Brook University
Stony Brook, New York

**Allen Wong, DDS, EdD, DABSCD**
Associate Professor, Department Dental
Practice
Director, Hospital Dentistry Program
Arthur A. Dugoni School of Dentistry
University of the Pacific
San Francisco, California

# Foreword

We live in an age where we count on our health care system to deliver the best scientific knowledge about the human body in the history of humanity. Every day, it seems, there's another breakthrough—a new treatment for cancer, a new less invasive surgery, a miracle drug, a computerized machine that can work wonders. Arrive at the doctor's office, and we expect to be amazed by the new, the technical, the cure.

But there is another element to medicine that is not new, but that is no less important: care. It is the language and the tradition of caring. It is, after all, caring that grounds medicine in the wisdom of the ages. Just as we count on the products of the laboratory to amaze us with new promises of life extended and improved, we also count on the human beings whom we meet in illness, or in an effort to preempt illness, to convey that most precious of human gifts: the gift of compassion, of empathy, of caring. No medicine is more powerful than caring.

Alas, for people with intellectual disabilities and development disabilities, the caring that we expect from medical and dental professionals has often been either lacking or openly denied. It is a sad fact that many health professionals, including dental professionals, shy away from treating patients with intellectual or developmental disabilities. Oftentimes, these professionals lack confidence and training for addressing the oral health needs of people with disabilities, even though it can be an incredibly rewarding experience for patients and providers. We are proud that since Special Olympics implemented the Healthy Athletes Program some 15 years ago nearly 1.4 million Special Olympics athletes have received free health screenings, including assessments, some direct treatment, education, and referrals for follow-up care. This has been through the generous donations of professional time and skills by more than a hundred thousand health professionals and students. The contributors to this textbook are among this esteemed group of caring professionals.

At Special Olympics, we see and treat thousands of athletes who have been routinely denied access to dental care their entire lives. As a result, these individuals often suffer tremendous pain from untreated dental conditions that have a detrimental effect on overall health. Based on our research, we believe that 39% of Special Olympics athletes have obvious untreated tooth decay and 29% are missing teeth. An inexcusable 15% of athletes are experiencing pain in their mouths due to dental problems on a regular basis. The clear message is simple: people with intellectual disabilities are facing a silent crisis of injustice in the health care system. For many, neither cure nor care is offered.

This is a crisis that can and must end, and happily, we have it within our power to end it. To do so, education is a critical first step. More than 50% of U.S. medical and dental school deans report that graduates of their programs are "not competent" to treat people with intellectual disabilities. If graduates of the world's best medical and dental institutions are not comfortable treating people with disabilities, we cannot expect them to provide quality care. But this gap in education can be closed, and this textbook will help close it. I hope *Dental Treatment for the Patient with a Developmental Disorder* becomes standard reading in dental training programs so that professionals can expand their practices and realize what an incredibly rewarding experience it is to make a difference in the life of a person with a disability.

With education comes confidence, and the source of our confidence today lies in the dedicated men and women who have contributed to this textbook. All have in their own way made it their life's work to bring justice to our fellow citizens with intellectual and developmental disabilities. Happily, they are each gifted scientists and health practitioners, so the research they offer in this book is of the highest value to the field. But equally happily, they each understand that a health care system that doesn't care about some is a health care system that doesn't care. And so each of them has been a leader of our "dignity revolution," matching their professional expertise with their human resolve to be agents of compassion and care for all.

That combination offers hope to each of us. And it is with that hope that we can all believe that someday very soon, all people with differences will knock on the doors of dentists and health care professionals the world over and be welcomed to the best in cure and care alike.

Timothy P. Shriver, PhD
Chairman & CEO of Special Olympics

# Preface

I have always sensed that "fear of the unknown" is what has kept many dental professionals from taking the leap and making a concerted effort to provide dental treatment and advocacy for people with developmental disorders. Perhaps the scariest thoughts in life are the "what-ifs." What if I do something wrong? What if something bad happens when I'm trying to do something good? What if I fail? What if I make a mistake?

My hope is that this textbook, with its unprecedented compilation of work from experts who have taken this leap and are practicing and teaching all over the world, will help new students, as well as long-standing practicing clinicians, feel more confident to go ahead and take that leap. The information provided should help wipe away the "fear of the unknown" factor and, at the least, help more dental professionals feel that they have the power to advocate for this patient population that needs them the most.

My passion for the creation of this textbook comes from what I have learned as both a dental hygienist and most importantly as a parent of a 12-year-old son with autism. He still today is not able to communicate with words effectively enough to ask for help, but he knows those people in his life who have been his greatest advocates and, without words, he expresses his gratitude to them every day. Imagine receiving that gift as a reward for your services.

Dr. Steven Perlman and I are honored to bring this compilation of work to the dental profession. We welcome your thoughts and feedback.

Karen A. Raposa, raposaredi@hotmail.com
Steven P. Perlman, sperlman@bu.edu

# Introduction

## The amazing tale of the three dentists, the cliff diver, and the avoidance of the mundane

Rick Rader, MD, FAAIDD

Before the young, idealistic dental health student got too far into this long-awaited text, I thought I could best serve the contributors as a "warm-up act" before the main act. I thought my role might be likened to the half-baked stand-up comedian opening up for Lady Gaga or Taylor Swift, except for the fact that you can't fast-forward through the preamble to the concert like you can these introductory pages. So I wanted to start with "so these three dentists walk into a bar and one of them, the short one, has a parrot on her shoulder..." But I can't because despite researching the exiting archives of over three and a half million jokes from over seventy countries, I was unable to unearth even one joke that showcased three dentists walking into a bar.

Often we see Oscar Wilde's antimimetic philosophy of "life imitates art" come to bear. So these three dentists walk into a bar; more specifically, they were out celebrating their twentieth graduation reunion. After graduation they all pursued different specialty arenas and it was great to finally be catching up. The first dentist shares that he has been practicing cosmetic dentistry in Boca Raton and life has been grand despite having trouble finding a decent mechanic for his Ferrari. The three clinked their shot glasses together in harmonious celebration. The second dentist followed with, "That sounds great. I've been practicing oral surgery with offices in the Hamptons and Manhattan," and that he has everything he had ever aspired to have. The three once again clinked their glasses in unison. The third dentist took a quick sip and shared that he had by some strange twist of fate practiced general dentistry in a large state developmental center, and when that closed he opened up his own practice in the community treating patients with intellectual and developmental disabilities; and that he had fulfilled his every dream as a dentist. The other two dentists half-heartedly held up their half-filled glasses, but instead of initiating a unified clinking of the glasses, the first one suffered, "Geez, sorry to hear that, what went wrong?" The second classmate followed by adding, "Couldn't you make it with real patients?"

Like I said, there are no jokes about three dentists walking into a bar, and this was certainly not an attempt to create the first one. This encounter, unfortunately, is not unique to dentists or dental hygienists who (somehow) found their professional pursuits satisfied by working with vulnerable patients and their families. The same stigma that is afforded to this marginalized, different and undervalued population is often applied to the dental professionals who both treat and advocate for them. Stigma by association.

And even though this was, admittedly, no joke, there is a punch line. The joke is on them, those classmates who ridiculed and invalidated the career choice of their classmate who found his way into the special needs arena.

I say the "joke is on them" because they failed to understand, appreciate, and value the richness of caring for and about individuals with complex disabilities. They unfortunately never got to experience the joy, the sheer unadulterated joy of practicing the purest form of dentistry. I doubt the joy they seemingly experienced on their Sunday drive in their Ferrari or on the rear deck of their Azimut yacht followed them into the office on Monday. That joy, the joy of caring for someone who has little to offer you except to authenticate your choice of entering the dental profession, is exactly what clinking glasses is all about.

Beyond the joy also lies the opportunity for an ongoing reinvigoration of the rewards of memorizing the Krebs cycle, of spending countless hours learning the obscure branches of facial nerves, and of poring over thousands of images in dental embryology, histology, and anatomy. The rewards of treating people with special needs also provide the rewards of getting to know people with special needs. They will challenge you, inspire you, rattle you, and comfort you. They will preserve in you that fragile hold of the real meaning of being a "healer," a feeling that was predictably diminished even before you completed your studies.

They will also transform your own self-image of what it means to be a dentist or a dental hygienist. Without realizing it you will cease to simply be a provider, a dental technocrat, to become an advocate. It is virtually impossible to invest in their lives without wanting to ensure that other opportunities (beyond dental care) are made available without undue obstacles or limitations. Thus your own organic initiation into the bicameral role of provider and advocate will be made possible by someone who asks for nothing in return for his or her facilitation.

Whether you become "that" dental professional in your community—the one who accepts, welcomes, and accommodates patients with intellectual and developmental disabilities or simply is exposed to them as part of your training, clerkships, or rotations—you will be better for having "been there, done that." While we need cosmetic dentists in Boca Raton as well as oral surgeons in the Hamptons, we also need individuals who have entered the dental profession with the realization that along with the skills, the rewards, and the respect comes a reverence for sheer, unadulterated caring. I am not necessarily referencing the need to care for others but rather the need to care for yourself, a need that can be enhanced by offering your skills to people who don't really care (or know) where you went to school and where in your class you graduated; people who simply care that you care.

So in essence, being a dentist or dental hygienist working in the special needs arena (or inviting several of them into your practice) with all the rewards and gifts it brings is quite possibly the most selfish thing you can do… way more selfish than a Ferrari or Azimut yacht. Go for it, indulge yourself. At least you won't have to worry about scratches and depreciation.

Finally, there is another aspect to caring for dental patients with special needs.

According to the official Current Dental Terminology listing there are 644 different procedures that are performed (at least coded for) by dentists. That number could be broken down into approximately fifty (unique) skill sets (drill, fill, measure, create, craft, align, inject, apply, remove) … stuff that is done over and over again.

While that number is hard to ascertain, there are only a certain number of "things" you can do to teeth, gums, bones, nerves, and soft tissue (I think that about covers most of the structures found in the oral cavity; write me if you can think of others for the next edition) in a mouth. By the time the dentist or dental hygienist is 5 years out of school, he or she has probably performed these finite number of procedures enough times that it becomes almost a commonplace occurrence. It's sad that an invasive, highly skilled procedure with little margin for error being performed on a living human being can become commonplace. But that is the nature of improving competency over time. In fact, the "commonplace" is not only a byproduct of competence but it's almost a necessary attainment. Highly technical procedures should always demand absolute concentration and focus, but by repetition they become almost mundane; nothing more than a "shoulder shrug" of excitement, a yawn. Many dentists report feelings of boredom, monotony, and indifference; the antithesis of what they experienced when they initially struggled to master complex procedures. They fondly remember the exhilaration of that first flawless extraction. If only they could recapture that. Most "bored" dentists have their complacency readjusted when they encounter a "difficult" or "complex" case. This usually translates into something unforeseen or unanticipated or something atypical happens. While this does indeed "rock their boat" and change the mundane to "all hands on deck" mode, it's not what dentists or hygienists welcome or wish. The antidote for the mundane dental day is to take a common procedure and provide a novel, unique, or challenging (without the drama and trauma of a procedure gone bad) "milieu." Enter the patient with an intellectual and developmental disability. A person who because of his or her challenges can take a "mundane" two and a half somersault dive in the pike position and increase its "degree of difficulty." Individuals, unforgettable individuals who often (not always) bring some baggage into your office can make the mundane a pleasure. They bring novel levels of communication, behaviors, somatosensory frazzles, neuromotor limitations, trust issues, self-stimulatory antics, hypersensitivities, negative past encounters with health providers (including dentists and hygienists), and difficulties processing who you are and what your intentions might be. While many dentists cite these as the reason they avoid "those people," for those who enjoy, embrace, and welcome a good midmorning challenge, the rewards are plentiful. The reason that not every dental professional accepts patients with special needs is the same reason that some divers prefer the springboard over the platform … and then you have the cliff divers—they abhor the mundane.

Dental professionals working in "special needs" prefer the cliff. The climb is worth the view.

# Overview: defining developmental disorders

## H. Barry Waldman, DDS, MPH, PhD and Steven P. Perlman, DDS, MScD, DHL (Hon)

It was not that long ago when children with developmental disabilities and adults with a range of disorders did not exist. We never saw them in our schools, movies, or communities. President Roosevelt may have had an attack of poliomyelitis, but everyone knew he had no problem standing and walking. At least it all seemed that way.

It took a long time to find out that tens of millions of youngsters and the not so young with a vast range of disabilities were concealed out of sight in institutions or in family homes. Somehow it was disgraceful, shameful, embarrassing, and a reflection on other family members to have a relative with some type of developmental or intellectual disability—except maybe a 95-year-old great-grandmother. Only later did we find out that the press and just about everyone in Washington was involved in the cover-up to ensure that the president of the country did not appear weak during the years of the Depression and World War II.

But that was the middle and the final decades of the twentieth century. In this second decade of the twenty-first century, we have learned that there are more than half a billion people in the world who are disabled as a consequence of mental, physical, and sensory impairment (United Nations 2010). "Disability is a complex phenomenon, reflecting an interaction between features of a person's body and features of the society in which he or she lives" (World Health Organization 2008). In the United States, there are more than fifty million individuals with developmental disabilities,

*Treating the Dental Patient with a Developmental Disorder*, First Edition.
Edited by Karen A. Raposa and Steven P. Perlman.
© 2012 John Wiley & Sons, Inc. Published 2012 by John Wiley & Sons, Inc.

complex medical problems, significant physical limitations, and a vast array of other conditions under the rubric of "disabilities" who live in local communities; many as a result of deinstitutionalization and mainstreaming them into community housing, education, and employment (U.S. Census Bureau 2010a).

The U.S. Census Bureau reported for 2006, among the total population:

- 5 years and over—6.8% had one disability. 8.3% had two or more disabilities.
- Five–15 years—536,400 had a sensory disability, almost 500,000 had a physical disability, and 2.8 million had an intellectual disability.
- Adults—37 million had a hearing disability, 21 million had a vision disability, and 15 million had a physical functioning disability. Specifically for seniors, 14.6 million had one or more disabilities (U.S. Census Bureau 2010a).

Among the non-institutionalized U.S. population 5 years and older:

- A larger number of females than males had physical, mental, and self-care disabilities—particularly in the older years, reflecting the greater longevity of females.
- A larger number of males than females had sensory disabilities (Table 1.1).

The number of persons with disabilities is projected to increase dramatically as the population 65 years and over reaches 1 in 5 residents during the next 2 decades (U.S. Census Bureau 2010b, 2010c). Media reports abound with references to the increasing numbers of older individuals with disabilities and government efforts to control the potential costs to service their mounting needs. By contrast, attention to the costs for youngsters with disabilities generally is centered on supportive education programs. Health financial issues, particularly during the years when youngsters enter adulthood, tend to be underreported.

It is estimated that the lifetime costs for all people with intellectual disabilities who were born in the United States in 2000 will total $51.2 billion (in 2003 dollars). These costs include both direct and indirect costs. Direct medical costs, including physician visits, prescription drugs, and inpatient hospital stays, account for 14% of these costs. Direct nonmedical expenses, such as home modifications and special education, make up 10% of the costs. Indirect costs, which include the value of lost wages when a person dies early, cannot work, or is limited in the amount or type of work that can be done, make up 70% of costs. These estimates do not include expenses such as hospital outpatient visits, emergency room visits, residential care, and family out-of-pocket expenses. The actual economic costs of intellectual disabilities are, therefore, even higher (CDC 2010e). Specifically, the average per capita society lifetime cost for individuals with autism through 66 years of age is $3.1 million (Ganz 2007).

**Table 1.1** Non-institutionalized U.S. residents (in thousands) with disabilities by gender and age: 2006 (U.S. Census Bureau 2010a).

|  | Male | Female |
|---|---|---|
| Sensory disabilities: | | |
| 5–15 yrs | 292 | 229 |
| 16–20 | 155 | 126 |
| 21–64 | 2,926 | 2,215 |
| 65–74 | 1,028 | 835 |
| 75+ | 1,674 | 2,347 |
| Total | 6,075 | 5,752 |
| Physical disabilities: | | |
| 5–15 yrs | 289 | 218 |
| 16–20 | 172 | 179 |
| 21–64 | 6,346 | 7,433 |
| 65–74 | 1,828 | 2,515 |
| 75+ | 2,346 | 4,453 |
| Total | 10,981 | 14,798 |
| Mental disabilities: | | |
| 5–15 yrs | 1,529 | 758 |
| 16–20 | 626 | 388 |
| 21–64 | 4,033 | 4,186 |
| 65–74 | 654 | 783 |
| 75+ | 1,053 | 1,915 |
| Total | 7,895 | 8,030 |
| Self-care disabilities: | | |
| 5–15 yrs | 240 | 148 |
| 16–20 | 89 | 66 |
| 21–64 | 1,835 | 2,197 |
| 65–74 | 455 | 677 |
| 75+ | 807 | 1,780 |
| Total | 3,426 | 4,868 |

# TYPES OF DISORDERS

This chapter will describe the more common developmental disorders in the literature today. However, it is important to note that there are literally hundreds that exist and hundreds that are yet to be identified.

## Autism spectrum disorders

Autism spectrum disorders (ASDs), also known as pervasive developmental disorders, are a group of developmental disorders defined by a significant impairment in social interaction and communication and by the presence of unusual behaviors and interests. Many individuals with ASD have atypical ways of learning, paying attention, or reacting to different sensations and stimuli. The assessment and learning abilities of youngsters and adults with ASD can vary from gifted to severely challenged. ASDs usually are diagnosed before age 3 and last throughout a person's life. ASDs occur in all racial, ethnic, and socioeconomic groups and are 4 times more likely to occur in boys than girls (CDC 2010a). "If 4 million children are born in the United States every year, approximately 24,000 of these children will eventually be diagnosed with ASD" (CDC 2010b).

The Centers for Disease Control and Prevention (CDC) conducts two nationally representative surveys in which parents are asked whether their child has ever received a diagnosis of autism. Estimates from these studies suggest that, as of 2003–2004, autism had been diagnosed in at least three hundred thousand children aged 4–17 years (CDC 2010d). "CDC estimates 1 in 88 children in United States has been identified as having an autism spectrum disorder" (CDC 2012).

Based upon these national studies and other CDC local studies, it is estimated that up to five hundred thousand individuals between the ages of 0 and 21 years have an autism spectrum disorder (Yeargin-Allsopp et al. 2003; Bertrand et al. 2005) (Table 1.2). A CDC study found that the rate

**Table 1.2** Prevalence of parent-reported autism among non-institutionalized children age 4–17 years (per 1,000 children) by selected demographic characteristics 2003–2004 (U.S. Census Bureau 2010a).

|  | NHIS* | NSCH* |
| --- | --- | --- |
| Gender: | | |
| Male | 8.8 | 8.5 |
| Female | 2.4 | 2.3 |
| Age (yrs): | | |
| 4–5 | 4.8 | 4.4 |
| 6–8 | 7.5 | 7.6 |
| 9–11 | 7.2 | 5.8 |
| 12–14 | 4.6 | 4.3 |
| 15–17 | 4.2 | 4.1 |
| Race/ethnicity: | | |
| Hispanic | 2.9 | 3.2 |
| White, non-Hispanic | 7.0 | 6.2 |
| Black, non-Hispanic | 5.2 | 5.8 |
| Highest level of education achieved by family member: | | |
| ≤ High school grad. | 4.0 | 4.1 |
| > High school grad. | 6.6 | 6.0 |
| Family income: | | |
| < 200% poverty level | 5.7 | 5.6 |
| ≥ 200% poverty level | | 7.1 |

*NHIS - National Health Interview Survey
NSCH - National Survey of Children's Health

among young children (3–10 years) was lower than the rate for intellectual disabilities but higher than the rates for cerebral palsy, hearing loss, and vision impairment.

More children are being classified as having an autism spectrum disorder, but it is unclear how much of this increase is due to changes in how one identifies and classifies people with ASDs or whether it is a true increase in prevalence (Shieve et al. 2006). By current standards, "the ASDs are the second most common serious developmental disability after mental retardation/intellectual impairment" (CDC 2010c).

The total number of children (3–22 years of age) with ASDs in a state is, to a great extent, a reflection of the variation in state populations. As of 2003, there were almost 25,000 youngsters with ASDs in California, almost 12,000 in Texas, and approximately 9,500 in New York. In addition, there were between 5,000 and more than 7,000 children with ASDs in 9 states, and between 1,000 and more than 4,000 children with ASDs in 21 states (Statemaster.com 2010).

Whether because of (1) better diagnosis, (2) a broader definition of autism, (3) a marked enlargement in the population of a particular state (e.g., Nevada), or (4) an actual increase in the numbers of individuals with ASDs, nationally between 1992 and 2003 there has been about a 2,560% increase in reported cases. These increases range from 23,300% in Ohio, 17,700% in Nevada, 16,200% in Wisconsin, 12,500% in Maryland, and 11,600% in New Hampshire, to between 1,000% and 5,000% in twenty-one states and less than 500% in eight states. There was a 1,086% increase in California (Table 1.3).

**Table 1.3** Cumulative growth of autism cases in children (ages 6–22 years) by state: 1992–2003 (Statemaster.com 2010).

|  | % increase |
| --- | --- |
| Ohio | 23,291 |
| Nevada | 17,720 |
| Wisconsin | 16,195 |
| Maryland | 12,529 |
| New Hampshire | 11,600 |

Between 1,000% and 5,000% increase (in decreasing order):
  Colorado, Arkansas, Minnesota, Illinois, Mississippi, Vermont, Nebraska, Montana, Kentucky, New Mexico, Idaho, Connecticut, Rhode Island, Alaska, Georgia, California, Oklahoma, Iowa, North Dakota, Guam, Maine, Kansas

Between 500% and 980% increase (in decreasing order):
  Wyoming, New Jersey, Utah, South Dakota, Arizona, Pennsylvania, Missouri, Texas, Alabama, South Carolina, Florida, Oregon, Hawaii, District of Columbia, Massachusetts, Virginia, Indiana

Between 40% and 472% increase (in decreasing order):
  Washington, Michigan, West Virginia, American Samoa, Northern Mariana Islands, North Carolina, Louisiana, Puerto Rico, Tennessee, New York, Delaware, U.S. Virgin Islands

National average = 2,560% increase

The number of children ages 3–22 with ASDs per 10,000 population in Oregon and Minnesota is about 4–5 times greater than the proportions in West Virginia, Montana, Oklahoma, Mississippi, New Mexico, and Colorado, as well as the Northern Mariana Islands, Puerto Rico, the U.S. Virgin Islands, and American Samoa (Statemaster.com 2010).

## Types of autism spectrum disorders

1.  Asperger syndrome: characterized by a greater or lesser degree of impairment in language and communication skills, as well as repetitive or restrictive patterns of thought and behavior. The most distinguishing symptom of Asperger syndrome is a child's obsessive interest in a single object or topic to the exclusion of any other. Unlike children with other types of autism, children with Asperger syndrome retain their early language skills (National Institute of Neurological Disorders and Stroke 2010c).
2.  Rett syndrome: characterized by normal early development followed by loss of purposeful use of the hands, distinctive body movements, slowed brain and head growth, gait abnormalities, seizures, and intellectual disabilities. It affects females almost exclusively (National Institute of Neurological Disorders and Stroke 2010b).
3.  Pervasive developmental disorder, not otherwise specified (PDD-NOS): encompasses cases where there is marked impairment of social interaction, communication, and/or stereotyped behavior patterns or interest (Yale Developmental Disabilities Clinic 2010b).
4.  Childhood disintegrative disorder: a rare condition that resembles autism but only after a relatively prolonged period (usually 2–4 years) of clearly normal development. Typically language, interest in the social environment, and often toileting and self-care abilities are lost, and there may be a general loss of interest in the environment (Yale Developmental Disabilities Clinic 2010a).
5.  Fragile X syndrome: a genetic condition involved in changes in part of the X chromosome. It is the most common form of inherited intellectual disability in males and a significant cause of intellectual disability in females. Fragile X syndrome is caused by a change in the FMR1 gene. A small section of the gene code (three letters only—CGG) is repeated on the fragile bottom area of the X chromosome. (The name "fragile X" was derived from the appearance of the X chromosome in a specialized tissue culture, because it looked like the end of the chromosome was broken.) The more repeats in the gene code, the more likely there is to be a problem. Normally, the FMR1 gene makes a protein needed for normal brain development. As a result of a defect in this gene, too little or none at all of the protein is produced. A male and female can both be affected, but because males have only one X chromosome, a fragile X is likely to affect them more severely (MedlinePlus 2010). Men pass the mutation only to their daughters. Their sons receive a Y chromosome, which

does not include the FMR1 gene. Fragile X syndrome occurs in approximately 1 in 4,000 males and 1 in 8,000 females (Genetics Home Reference 2010).

When the gene shuts down in people with fragile X syndrome, the result is that brain cells do not communicate normally and cause a form of hyperactive brain activity, a form common in many autism spectrum disorders. Compounds exist that dampen these effects. Studies are under way using lithium to intervene with autism and fragile X syndrome symptoms (Fraxa Research Foundation 2010).

6. Savant syndrome: not a recognized medical diagnosis. It is a rare condition in which people with developmental disorders have one or more areas of expertise, ability, or brilliance that are in contrast with the individual's overall limitations. About half of persons with savant syndrome have autistic disorder, while the others have another developmental disability, intellectual disability, brain injury, or disease. Savant syndrome is 6 times more frequent in males than females (Savant syndrome 2010).

## Down syndrome

Down syndrome is a set of mental and physical symptoms that result from having an extra copy of chromosome 21 (called trisomy 21), which affects brain and body development. While individuals with Down syndrome may have some physical and mental features in common, the signs can range from mild to severe. Usually mental and physical developments are slower than in those individuals without the condition. IQs range in the mild to profound range of intellectual disability. Language and physical motor development may be delayed or slow. Common physical signs include:

- Flat face with an upward slant to the eyes, short neck, and abnormally shaped ears.
- Deep crease in the palm of the hand.
- White spots on the iris of the eye.
- Poor muscle tone, loose ligaments.
- Small hands and feet.

There are a variety of other health conditions that often are seen, including:

- Congenital heart disease—30–50% have heart defects at birth.
- Hearing loss and eye problems (mostly due to cataracts). These changes tend to occur 20–30 years before other persons in the general population.
- Intestinal problems, such as blocked small bowel or esophagus—8–12% have gastrointestinal tract abnormalities at birth.
- Celiac disease.
- Thyroid dysfunction.

- Skeletal problems.
- Dementia—similar to Alzheimer's disease (National Institute of Child Health and Human Development 2010; National Down Syndrome Congress 2010).

Down syndrome is the most commonly inherited form of learning disability. In developed countries it accounts for 12–15% of the population with learning disabilities (Bittles & Glasson 2004). The chance of having a baby with Down syndrome increases as a woman gets older—from about 1 in 1,250 for a woman who becomes pregnant at age 25, to about 1 in 100 for a woman who becomes pregnant at age 40. But most babies with Down syndrome are born to women under 35 years because of the fact that younger women have more babies. Parents who already have a child with Down syndrome or who have abnormalities in their own chromosome 21 are also at higher risk for having a baby with Down syndrome (National Institute of Child Health and Human Development 2010). Approximately 5,000 children with Down syndrome are born each year in this country. The condition is not related to race, nationality, religion, or socio-economic status (National Down Syndrome Congress 2010). There are presently more than 350,000 people in the United States with this genetic condition (National Down Syndrome Society 2010). Advances in medical treatments have greatly improved the life expectancy of people with Down syndrome, with the majority living past age 55 (Harvard Medical School Consumer Health Information 2010).

## Attention deficit hyperactivity disorder

Attention deficit hyperactivity disorder (ADHD) is a neurobehavioral developmental disorder that affects about 3–5% of the world's population. It is thought to be caused by problems in the regulation of two neurotransmitters, dopamine and norepinephrine, which are believed to play an important role in the ability to focus and pay attention to tasks. "Genetic research strongly suggests that ADHD tends to run in families and that 55% of diagnosed adults have one or more children with ADHD" (Dodson 2008). It usually presents itself during childhood and is characterized by a persistent pattern of impulsiveness and inattention, with or without a component of hyperactivity (Attention-deficit hyperactivity disorder 2010).

In 2006, an estimated 4.5 million school-age children (5–17 years of age) had been diagnosed with ADHD and 4.6 million children with learning disorder (LD). Past estimates of the prevalence of ADHD and LD have varied, in part, because of differences in the criteria used for identifying these conditions and the variations in the population that were selected for study (Pastor & Reuben 2008). A recent national survey of special education students showed that youngsters with ADHD are a rapidly growing group of students within special education programs (Schnoes et al. 2006). Though previously regarded as a childhood diagnosis, studies have shown that

ADHD may continue through adulthood, though generally with a reduction in hyperactivity that may adversely affect day-to-day vocational, social, and family functioning (Attention-deficit hyperactivity disorder 2010). Between 10% and 60% of individuals diagnosed in childhood with ADHD continue to meet the diagnostic criteria in adulthood. As they mature, adolescents and adults with ADHD are likely to develop coping mechanisms to compensate for their impairment (Elia et al. 1999; Gentile et al. 2006; Therapeutics letter 2008).

## Tic disorder

Tic disorder is a problem in which a part of the body moves repeatedly, quickly, suddenly, and uncontrollably. Tics can occur in any body part, such as the face, shoulders, hands, or legs. They can be stopped voluntarily for brief periods. Sounds that are made involuntarily (such as throat clearing) are called vocal tics. Most tics are mild and hardly noticeable. However, in some cases they are frequent and severe, and they can affect many areas of a child's life.

The most common tic disorder is called "transient tic disorder" and may affect up to 10% of children during the early school years. Teachers or others may notice the tics and wonder if the child is under stress or "nervous." Transient tics go away by themselves. Some may get worse with anxiety, tiredness, and some medications. Some tics do not go away. Tics that last 1 year or more are called "chronic tics." Chronic tics affect less than 1% of children and may be related to a special, more unusual tic disorder called Tourette's disorder.

Children with Tourette's disorder have both body and vocal tics (throat clearing). Some tics disappear by early adulthood and some continue. Children with Tourette's disorder may also have problems with attention and learning disabilities. They may act impulsively and/or develop obsessions and compulsions. Sometimes people with Tourette's disorder may blurt out obscene words, insult others, or make obscene gestures or movements. They cannot control these sounds and movements and should not be blamed for them. Punishment by parents, teasing by classmates, and scolding by teachers will not help the child to control the tics but will hurt the child's self-esteem and increase his or her distress (American Academy of Child and Adolescent Psychiatry 2010).

## Dyspraxia

Dyspraxia is a neurological disorder of motor coordination usually apparent in childhood that manifests as difficulty in thinking out, planning out, and executing planned movements or tasks. Dyspraxia is a variable condition; it manifests in different ways at different ages. It may impair physical, intellectual, emotional, social, language, and/or sensory development. Dyspraxia is often subdivided into two types: developmental dyspraxia and verbal dyspraxia. Symptoms of the dyspraxia typically appear in childhood, anywhere from infancy to adolescence, and can persist into adult years. Other disorders such as dyslexia, learning disabilities, and attention deficit disorder often co-occur in children with dyspraxia. Estimates of the prevalence of developmental coordination disorder are approximately 6% in children aged 5–11. Some reports indicate a higher prevalence in the 10–20% range. Males are 4 times more likely than females to have dyspraxia. In some cases, the disorder may be familial (Answers.com 2010b).

## Cerebral palsy

Cerebral palsy refers to any one of a number of neurological disorders that appear in infancy or early childhood and permanently affect body movement and muscle coordination but don't worsen over time. Even though cerebral palsy affects muscle movement, it isn't caused by problems in the muscles or nerves. It is caused by abnormalities in parts of the brain that control muscle movements. The majority of children with cerebral palsy are born with it, although it may not be detected until months or years later. The early signs of cerebral palsy usually appear before a child reaches 3 years of age. The most common are a lack of muscle coordination when performing voluntary movements (ataxia); stiff or tight muscles and exaggerated reflexes (spasticity); walking with one foot or leg dragging; walking on the toes, a crouched gait, or a "scissored" gait; and muscle tone that is either too stiff or too flaccid. A small number of children have cerebral palsy as the result of brain damage in the first few months or years of life, brain infections such as bacterial meningitis or viral encephalitis, or head injury from a motor vehicle accident, a fall, or child abuse. It is estimated that about 764,000 children and adults in the United States have one or more of the symptoms of cerebral palsy. Currently, about 8,000 babies and infants are diagnosed with the condition each year. In addition, some 1,200–1,500 preschool-age children are recognized each year to have cerebral palsy (National Institute of Neurological Disorders and Stroke 2010; United Cerebral Palsy 2010).

## Intellectual disabilities

An intellectual disability (ID) is characterized both by a significantly below-average score on a test of mental ability or intelligence and by limitations in the ability to function in areas of daily life, such as communication, self-care, and getting along in social situations and school activities. ID is the most common developmental disorder. Approximately 350 million people throughout the world are affected by ID. (Intellectual disability is sometimes referred to as a cognitive disability or mental retardation.)

ID occurs in 2.5–3% of the general population. About 6–7.5 million individuals with ID live in the United States. ID begins in childhood or adolescence before the age of 18. In most cases, it persists throughout adulthood. Specifically, a diagnosis of ID is made if an individual has an intellectual functioning level well below average and significant limitations in two or more adaptive skill areas. Intellectual functioning level is defined by standardized tests that measure the ability to reason in terms of mental age (intelligence quotient or IQ). Intellectual disability is defined as IQ score below 70–75. Adaptive skills are the skills needed for daily life. Such skills include the ability to produce and understand language (communication); home-living skills; use of community resources; health, safety, leisure, self-care, and social skills; self-direction; functional academic skills (reading, writing, and arithmetic); and work skills.

Intellectual disability varies in severity:

- Mild—approximately 85% of the population with ID is in the mild category. Their IQ score ranges from 50 to 75, and they can often acquire academic skills up to the 6th-grade level. They can become fairly self-sufficient and in some cases live independently, with community and social support.
- Moderate—about 10% of the population with ID is considered moderately retarded. These individuals have IQ scores ranging from 35 to 55. They can carry out work and self-care tasks with moderate supervision. They typically acquire communication skills in childhood and are able to live and function successfully within the community in a supervised environment such as a group home.
- Severe—about 3–4% of the population with ID is severely affected. These individuals have IQ scores of 20–40. They may master very basic self-care skills and some communication skills. Many affected individuals are able to live in a group home.
- Profound—only 1–2% of the population with ID is profoundly affected. These individuals have IQ scores under 20–25. They may be able to develop basic self-care and communication skills with appropriate support and training. Their condition is often caused by an accompanying neurological disorder. The profoundly affected need a high level of structure, supervision, and care.

It is estimated that among children 6–21 years in the United States, one-half million have some level of intellectual disability and are served in school under the Individuals with Disabilities Education Act (CDC 2010f; International Association for the Scientific Study of Intellectual Disabilities 2010; U.S. Department of Education 2010; Answers.com 2010a).

## Visual, hearing, and speech disabilities

Among individuals 15 years and older, 6 million have some sight difficulties, 6.8 million have hearing difficulties, and 2.1 million have speech difficulties. The prevalence of each of these disabilities increases with age. Similarly,

**Table 1.4** Prevalence of sight, hearing, and speech disabilities among individuals 15 years and older: 2005 (numbers in millions; Brault 2010).

|  | 15 yrs+ | | 65 yrs+ | |
| --- | --- | --- | --- | --- |
|  | # | % | # | % |
| Sight: | | | | |
|   Some difficulty | 6.0 | 2.6 | 2.5 | 7.3% |
|   Severe | 1.8 | 0.8 | 1.0 | 2.8 |
| Hearing: | | | | |
|   Some difficulty | 6.8 | 3.0 | 3.4 | 9.7 |
|   Severe | 1.0 | 0.4 | 0.5 | 1.5 |
| Speech: | | | | |
|   Some difficulty | 2.1 | 0.9 | 0.6 | 1.8 |
|   Severe | 0.4 | 0.2 | 0.1* | 0.3 |

*Limitation on confidence of number.
Note: Numbers have been rounded to nearest hundred thousand.

the prevalence of severe disabilities for vision, hearing, and speech increases with age (Table 1.4).

## Learning disabilities

It is believed that learning disabilities affecting 4.6 million children are caused by a difficulty with the nervous system that affects receiving, processing, or communicating information. They may also run in families. Some children with learning disabilities are also hyperactive; they are unable to sit still, easily distracted, and have a short attention span. Signs of LD may include:

- Difficulty understanding and following instructions.
- Trouble remembering what someone just told him or her.
- Fails to master reading, spelling, writing, and/or math skills.
- Difficulty distinguishing right from left; difficulty identifying words or a tendency to reverse letters, words, or numbers (e.g., confusing 25 with 52, "b" with "d," or "on" with "no"). The "right-left complexity" is referred to as dyslexia, a language-based learning disability that results in people having difficulties with specific language skills, particularly reading.
- Lacking coordination in walking, sports, or small activities such as holding a pencil or tying a shoelace.
- Easily loses or misplaces homework, schoolbooks, or other items.
- Cannot understand the concept of time; is confused by "yesterday, today and tomorrow" (American Academy of Child and Adolescent Psychiatry 2010).

There are a variety of learning disorders. Some cause problems or difficulties with language (both written and spoken), reading, writing, math, attention, and control. Learning disabilities are not due to mental or emotional problems. Learning disabilities are also not associated with someone having less of an economic or social advantage than someone else. At least 10% of the population has one or more learning disabilities. In special education classrooms, almost 40% of the students have a learning disability. Many more are probably affected throughout the world but have not been diagnosed yet (University of Phoenix 2010).

## Psychiatric disorders

There are over three hundred different psychiatric disorders listed in the *Diagnostic and Statistical Manual of Mental Disorders* (DSM-IV), including generalized anxiety, depression, bipolar disorder, schizophrenia, mood, sleep, and a seeming endless array of personal disorders. With continued research, more are named every year and some disorders are removed or recategorized. An estimated almost 16 million non-institutionalized U.S. residents 5 years and older have some form of mental disability (All Psych Online 2010) (Table 1.1).

## Cleft lip and palate

Cleft lip and palate is the nonfusion of the body's natural structures that form before birth. One in 700 children born have a cleft lip and/or a palate. Craniofacial defects such as cleft lip and cleft palate are among the most common of all birth defects. The average annual number of cleft palate cases is 2,567; cleft lip with or without cleft palate cases is 4,209. They can occur as an isolated condition or may be one component of an inherited disease or syndrome. A cleft lip or palate can be surgically treated soon after birth. The lifetime cost of treating the children born each year with cleft lip or cleft palate is estimated to be $697 million (National Institute of Dental and Craniofacial Research 2010).

## Spina bifida

Spina bifida is among the most common permanently disabling birth defect in the United States. It occurs when the spine of a baby fails to close during the first month of pregnancy. Some vertebrae overlying the spinal cord are not fully formed and remain unfused and open. Spina bifida can be surgically closed after birth, but this does not restore normal function to the affected part of the spinal cord. If the opening is large enough, this allows a portion of the spinal cord to protrude through the opening in the bones. The incidence of spina bifida can be decreased by up to 75% when daily folic acid supplements are taken prior to conception.

The conservative estimate is that there are 166,000 living with spina bifida in the United States. The average total lifetime cost to society for each infant born with spina bifida is approximately $532,000 per child. This estimate is only an average, and for many children the total cost may be well above $1 million. Estimated total annual medical care and surgical costs for persons with spina bifida in the United States exceed $200 million.

Risk factors for neural tube defects (NTDs) include:

- A previous NTD-affected pregnancy increases a woman's chance to have another NTD-affected pregnancy by approximately 20 times.
- Maternal insulin-dependent diabetes.
- Use of certain anti-seizure medication (valproic acid/Depakene, and carbamazapine/Tegretol).
- Medically diagnosed obesity.
- High temperatures in early pregnancy (i.e., prolonged fevers and hot tub use).
- Race/ethnicity NTDs are more common among white women than black women and more common among Hispanic women than non-Hispanic women.
- Lower socio-economic status (Spina Bifida Association 2010).

## Fetal alcohol syndrome (fetal alcohol spectrum disorders)

Fetal alcohol spectrum disorders (FASDs) affect an estimated forty thousand infants each year in the United States—more than spina bifida, Down syndrome, and muscular dystrophy combined. Alcohol use during pregnancy is the leading known preventable cause of intellectual disability and birth defects in this country. While there is no cure for FASD, it is 100% preventable. It is believed to be the third most common cause of intellectual disability worldwide. Alcohol causes neurological damage and cell loss in the fetal brain, on which it acts as a toxin.

Defects caused by prenatal exposure to alcohol have been identified in virtually every part of the body, including brain, face, eyes, ears, heart, kidneys, and bones. Alcohol sets in motion many processes at different sites in the developing fetus just a few weeks after conception when many women are unaware that they are pregnant and/or are now aware of consequences to the embryo.

Signs of fetal alcohol syndrome may include:

- Distinctive facial features, including small eyes, an exceptionally thin upper lip, a short, upturned nose, and a smooth skin surface between the nose and upper lip.
- Heart defects.
- Deformities of joints, limbs, and fingers.
- Slow physical growth before and after birth.
- Vision difficulties or hearing problems.

- Small head circumference and brain size.
- Poor coordination.
- Sleep problems.
- Intellectual disability and delayed development.
- Learning disorders.
- Abnormal behavior, such as a short attention span, hyperactivity, poor impulse control, extreme nervousness, and anxiety.

## SUMMARY

It is difficult to comprehend the full impact of individuals with disabilities on our individual communities and the efforts required by health and social service providers, educational institutions, and the families of individuals with developmental disorders when we are confronted with the facts that:

- There are more than fifty million individuals with disabilities in our nation.
- 12.8% of the adult U.S. population (21–64 years) and 40.6% of the population 65 years and over have a seemingly infinite series of disabilities.

Nationwide data actually mask the reality of the wide variations in different areas and communities of the country. For example, the proportion of the adult population (21–64 years) with a disability ranges from 9.3% in New Jersey to 22.4% in West Virginia (Henry J. Kaiser Family Foundation 2010; U.S. Census Bureau 2010d) (Table 1.5).

## ABUSE AND NEGLECT OF PEOPLE WITH DEVELOPMENTAL DISABILITIES

Since this chapter serves as an overview of the category of developmental disorders, it would not be complete without mentioning the potential pain and suffering that many of these patients may endure in their lifetimes. It is difficult for us to conceive of anyone abusing individuals who already are compromised with developmental disabilities. It seems beyond belief that the literature is replete with studies that indicate that there are substantial increases in the risk of abuse for children and adults with disabilities. We tend to mask the unspeakable when we consider the "dirty secret" of abuse and neglect of children, young adults, and the elderly. The reality, however, is that maltreatment of individuals with (and without) developmental disabilities is all too real, especially for persons with disabilities, and all too often the perpetrator may be a caregiver or family member.

**Table 1.5** Percentage of adult population aged 21–64 years who reported a disability, 2007 (Kaiser Family Foundation 2010).

| | |
|---|---|
| United States | 12.8% |
| 1. New Jersey | 9.3% |
| 2. North Dakota | 10.1% |
| 3. Illinois | 10.3% |
| 4. Minnesota | 10.3% |
| 5. Connecticut | 10.4% |
| 6. Utah | 10.4% |
| 7. Hawaii | 10.7% |
| 8. Colorado | 10.8% |
| 9. California | 10.9% |
| 10. Maryland | 10.9% |
| 11. Nebraska | 10.9% |
| 12. Virginia | 11.1% |
| 13. Nevada | 11.2% |
| 14. New Hampshire | 11.3% |
| 15. Wisconsin | 11.3% |
| 16. Massachusetts | 11.4% |
| 17. New York | 11.7% |
| 18. District of Columbia | 11.8% |
| 19. Arizona | 12.0% |
| 20. Kansas | 12.0% |
| 21. Florida | 12.1% |
| 22. Delaware | 12.2% |
| 23. Texas | 12.2% |
| 24. Iowa | 12.4% |
| 25. Idaho | 12.6% |
| 26. Georgia | 12.7% |
| 27. South Dakota | 12.7% |
| 28. Vermont | 13.2% |
| 29. Montana | 13.5% |
| 30. Indiana | 13.6% |
| 31. Wyoming | 13.7% |
| 32. Pennsylvania | 13.8% |
| 33. Oregon | 13.9% |
| 34. Washington | 14.0% |
| 35. Ohio | 14.1% |
| 36. Rhode Island | 14.2% |
| 37. Michigan | 14.4% |
| 38. New Mexico | 14.5% |
| 39. North Carolina | 14.9% |
| 40. Alaska | 15.0% |
| 41. Missouri | 15.0% |
| 42. South Carolina | 15.1% |
| 43. Louisiana | 16.2% |
| 44. Tennessee | 16.8% |
| 45. Oklahoma | 17.3% |

**Table 1.5**   (cont'd)

| | |
|---|---|
| 46. Maine | 18.1% |
| 47. Arkansas | 19.0% |
| 48. Alabama | 19.3% |
| 49. Kentucky | 19.5% |
| 50. Mississippi | 19.5% |
| 51. West Virginia | 22.4% |

This information was reprinted with permission from the Henry J. Kaiser Family Foundation. The Kaiser Family Foundation, a leader in health policy analysis, health journalism, and communication, is dedicated to filling the need for trusted, independent information on the biggest health issues facing our nation and its people. The foundation is a nonprofit private operating foundation based in Menlo Park, California.

## Numbers

Compared to the general population of children, children with disabilities are 3.4 times more likely to be abused or neglected. They are 3.8 times more likely to be neglected, 3.8 times more likely to be physically abused, 3.1 times more likely to be sexually abused, and 3.9 times more likely to be emotionally abused (Sullivan & Knutson 2000).

People with disabilities are abused sexually mostly by caregivers whether it is the family or other disability service providers; specifically, 15–25% of the perpetrators of sexual abuse are natural family members, 15% are acquaintances and neighbors, 30% are disability service providers, and 0–5% are strangers (Wolberg 1994).

Approximately one million elderly Americans are physically abused each year, where the majority of the victims are female (Brunet 2011).

Maltreatment may include:

- Physical abuse—blunt trauma, burns with cigarettes, the use of knives, guns, and/or just about any of a seemingly endless list of objects.
- Sexual abuse—including completed and attempted vaginal, oral, and anal intercourse, cunnilingus, analingus, genital fondling, digital and foreign object penetration.
- Neglect—including physical and medical neglect, abandonment, inadequate supervision, inadequate nurturing/affection, refusal or delay of psychological care.
- Emotional and verbal abuse, lack of supportive and caring environment, and alcohol addictive abuse.

Contributing factors: the individual with a disability may be regarded as a source of embarrassment, and may symbolize "punishment" for the family. The family member with a disability:

- Alters family patterns, roles and routines in particular stressful ways, which may exceed family member's capacities and result in an abusive reaction.

- May strain housing and employment arrangements and family resources (including financial, socio-economic, and social resources), which in turn may impact on marital and general family relationships.
- May require unexpected and significant support at the time of other needs and wants of the family.
- May need services and support for an extended indeterminate period of time (Waldman et al. 1999).

## Perspective of the dental team

The dentist, dental hygienist, and staff members are in a position to recognize instances of physical, emotional, and sexual abuse, failure to thrive, intentional drugging or poisoning, and health (medical and dental) and safety neglect. In the case of children (and adults with diminished intellectual ability), the health professional's legal responsibility requires that even a suspicion of abuse must be reported to the proper authorities. Failure to do so may place the practitioner in legal jeopardy for failure to ensure the safety of the abused individual.

The reality is that health practitioners will be called upon to provide needed services on an individual basis for the hundreds or thousands of individuals with developmental disorders in their communities. It is from this perspective that the following chapters are presented.

# REFERENCES

All Psych Online. (2010). Psychiatric disorders. Accessed March 6, 2010, from http://allpsych.com/disorders/index.html.

American Academy of Child and Adolescent Psychiatry. (2010). Children with learning disabilities. Accessed March 6, 2010, from http://www.aacap.org/cs/root/facts_for_families/children_with_learning_disabilities.

Answers.com. (2010a). Mental retardation. Accessed March 5, 2010, from http://www.answers.com/topic/mental-retardation.

———. (2010b). Neurological disorders: Dyspraxia. Accessed March 3, 2010, from http:/www.answers.com/topic/dyspraxia.

Asa R. (2010). Special needs: Treating patients with fetal alcohol spectrum disorders. AGD Impact (online) 2010 (September):26–34.

Attention-deficit hyperactivity disorder. (2010). Wikipedia. Accessed March 1, 2010, from http://en.wikipedia.org/wiki/Attention-Deficit_Hyperactivity_Disorder.

Bertrand J, Mars A, Boyle C, et al. (2005). Prevalence of autism in a United States population: The Brick Township, New Jersey, investigation. *Pediatrics* 44:557–564.

Bittles AH, Glasson EJ. (2004). Clinical, social, and ethical implications of changing life expectancy in Down syndrome. *Developmental Medicine and Child Neurology* 46:282–286.

Brault MW. (2008). Census Bureau. Current Population Reports. Americans with Disabilities. Accessed March 6, 2010, from http://www.census.gov/prod/2008pubs/p70-117.pdf.

Brunet M. (2011). Troubles facing disabled and elderly women. Accessed March 23, 2011, from http://www.ehow.com/info_7808019_troubles-facing-disabled-elderly-women.html.

Centers for Disease Control and Prevention (CDC). (2010a). Autism. Accessed March 4, 2010, from http://twww.cdc.gov/ncbddd/autism.

———. (2010b). Autism: How common are autism spectrum disorders (ASD)? Accessed February 26, 2010, from http://www.cdc.gov/ncbddd/autism/asd_common.htm.

———. (2010c). Autism: What are the symptoms? Accessed March 1, 2010, from http://www.cdc.gov/ncbddd/autism/asd_symptoms.htm.

———. (2010d). Autism: What causes ASDs and is there a treatment? Accessed March 1, 2010, from http://www.cdc.gov/ncbddd/autism/asd_treatments.htm.

———. (2010e). Developmental disabilities: Intellectual disability. Accessed February 19, 2010, from http://www.cddc.gov/ncbddd/dd/mr4.htm.

———. (2010f). Intellectual disability. Accessed March 5, 2010, from http://www.cdc.gov/ncbddd/dd/ddmr.htm.

———. (2012). CDC estimates 1 in 88 children in United States has been identified as having an autism spectrum disorder. http://www.cdc.gov/media/releases/2012/p0329_autism_disorder.html

Dodson W. (2008). ADAD: Not just a childhood disorder. *EP Magazine* 38(10): 74–75.

Elia J, Ambrosini PJ, Rapoport JL. (1999). Treatment of attention-deficit-hyperactive disorder. *New England Journal of Medicine* 340:780–788.

Fraxa Research Foundation. (2010). Finding a cure for Fragile X. Accessed March 9, 2010, from http://www.fraxa.org/research_summaryFindings.aspx.

Ganz ML. (2007). The lifetime distribution of the incremental societal costs of autism. *Archives of Pediatric and Adolescent Medicine* 161:343–349.

Genetics Home Reference. (2010). Fragile X syndrome. Accessed March 10, 2010, from http://ghr.nlm.nih.gov/condition=fragilexsundrome.

Gentile JP, Atiq R, Gillig PM. (2006). Diagnosis, differential diagnosis, and medication management. *Psychiatry* 3:24–30.

Harvard Medical School Consumer Health Information. (2010). Down syndrome. Accessed March 4, 2010, from http://www.intelihealth.com/IH/ihtIH/WSIHW000/9339/9844.html.

Henry J. Kaiser Family Foundation, statehealthfacts.org. (2010). Percentage of adult population aged 21–64 years who reported a disability, 2008. Data source: Disability statistics from the American Community Survey (ACS). Ithaca, NY: Cornell University Rehabilitation Research and Training Center on Disability Demographics and Statistics (StatsRRTC). Accessed March 18, 2010, from http://www.disabilitystatistics.org.

International Association for the Scientific Study of Intellectual Disabilities. (2010). Aging and intellectual disabilities. Accessed March 5, 2010, from http://ddas.vt.gov/ddas-publications/publications-dementia/publications-dementia-documents/fs-aging-intellectual-disabilities.

Mayo Clinic.com. (2010). Fetal alcohol syndrome. Accessed November 9, 2010, from http://www.mayoclinic.com/health/fetal-alcohol-syndrome/DS00184/DSECTION=symptoms.

MedlinePlus. (2010). Fragile X syndrome. Accessed March 9, 2010, from http://www.nlm.nih.gov/medlineplus/ency/article/001668.htm.

National Down Syndrome Congress. (2010). Facts about Down syndrome. Accessed March 5, 2010, from http://www.ndsccenter.org/resources/package3.php.

National Down Syndrome Society. (2010). Topic information. Accessed March 5, 2010, from http://www.ndss.org/index.php?option=com_content&task=view&id=1812&Itemid=95.

National Institute of Child Health and Human Development. (2010). Down syndrome. Accessed March 5, 2010, from http://www.nichd.nih.gov/health/topics/Down_Syndrome.cfm.

National Institute of Dental and Craniofacial Research. (2010). Cleft lip and cleft palate. Accessed May 6, 2010, from http://www.nidcr.nih.gov/DataStatistics/FindDataByTopic/CraniofacialBirthDefects/PrevalenceCleft+LipCleftPalate.htm.

National Institute of Neurological Disorders and Stroke. (2010a). Cerebral palsy information page. Accessed March 5, 2010, from http://www.ninds.nih.gov/disorders/cerebral_palsy/cerebral_palsy.htm.

———. (2010b). Rett syndrome fact sheet. Accessed March 8, 2010, from http://www.ninds.nih.gov/disorders/rett/detail_rett.htm.

———. (2010c). What is Asperger syndrome? Accessed March 8, 2010, from http://www.ninds.nih.gov/disorders/asperger/asperger.htm.

Pastor PN, Reuben CA. (2008). Diagnosed attention deficit hyperactivity disorder and learning disability: United States, 2004–2006 (Vital Health Statistics, Series 10, No. 237). Hyattsville, MD: National Center for Health Statistics.

Savant syndrome. (2010). Wikipedia. Accessed March 3, 2010, from http://en.wikipedia.org/wiki/Savant_syndrome.

Schnoes C, Reid R, Wagner M, Marder C. (2006). ADHD among students receiving special education services: A national survey. *Exceptional Children* 72:483–496.

Shieve LA, Rice C, Boyle C, et al. (2006). Mental health in the United States: Parental report of diagnosed autism in children aged 4–17 years—United States, 2003–2004. *Morbidity and Mortality Weekly Report* 55:481–486.

Spina Bifida Association. (2010). Facts. Accessed March 6, 2010, from http://www.spinabifidaassociation.org/site/c.liKWL7PLLrF/b.2642297/k.5F7C/Spina_Bifida_Association.htm.

Statemaster.com. (2010). Health statistics: Number of children with autism by state. Accessed March 5, 2010, from http://www.statemaster.com.

Sullivan PM, Knutson JF. (2000). Maltreatment and disabilities: A population-based epidemiological study. *Child Abuse and Neglect* 24(10):1257–1273.

Therapeutics Letter. (2008). What is the evidence for using CNS stimulants to treat ADHD in children? March–May 2008. Accessed March 9, 2010, from http://

ti.ubc.ca/newsletter/what-evidence-using-cns-stimulants-treat-adhd-children).

United Cerebral Palsy. (2010). Cerebral palsy: Facts and figures. Accessed March 5, 2010, from http://www.ucp.org/ucp_generaldoc.cfm/1/9/37/37-37/447.

United Nations. (2010). World programme of action concerning disabled persons. Accessed March 3, 2010, from http://www.un.org/esa.socdev/enable/diswpa01.htm.

University of Phoenix. (2010). Most learning disabilities. Accessed March 6, 2010, from http://www.essortment.com/all/commonlearning_rnmz.htm.

U.S. Census Bureau. (2010a). Disability. Accessed March 3, 2010, from http://www.census.gov/hhes/www/disability/data_title.htm.

———. (2010b). Disability characteristics: 2006 American Community Survey (S1801). Accessed March 3, 2010, from http://factfinder.census.gov.

———. (2010c). Interim projections: Population under 18 years and 65 and older: 2000, 2010 and 2030. Accessed March 3, 2010, from http://www.census.gov/population/www/projections/projectsagesex.htm.

———. (2010d). Table S0103. Population 65 years and over in the United States—Data Set: 2007 American Community Survey 1-year estimates. Survey: American Community Survey Web site. Accessed March 7, 2010, from http://factfinder.census.gov/servlet/STTable?_bm=y&-qr_name=ACS_2007_1YR_G00_S0103&-geo_id=01000US&-ds_name=ACS_2007_1YR_G00_&-_lang=en&-format=&-CONTEXT=st.

U.S. Department of Education. Office of Special Education. (2010). Accessed March 10, 2010, from http://www/ideadata.org/index.html.

Waldman HB, Swerdloff M, Perlman SP. (1999). A "dirty secret": The abuse of children with disabilities. *Journal of Dentistry for Children* 66(3):197–202.

Wolberg G. (1994). Violence and abuse in the lives of people with disabilities. Accessed March 23, 2011, from http://www.bioethicsanddisability.org/violence.html.

World Health Organization. (2008). Disabilities. Accessed June 20, 2008, from http://www.who.int/topics/disabilities/en.

Yale Developmental Disabilities Clinic. (2010a). Childhood disintegrative disorder. Accessed March 4, 2010, from http://www.med.yale.edu/chldstdy/autism/cdd.html.

———. (2010b). Pervasive developmental disorder—not otherwise specified (PDD-NOS). Accessed March 3, 2010, from http://www.med.yale.edu/chldstdy/autism/pddnos.html.

Yeargin-Allsopp M, Rice C, Karapurkar T, et al. (2003). Prevalence of autism in a U.S. metropolitan area. *Journal of the American Medical Association* 289:49–55.

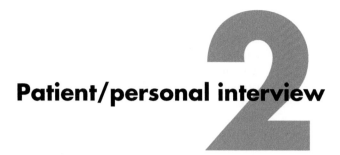

# Patient/personal interview

### Maureen Romer, DDS, MPA, FADPD, DABSCD

## INTRODUCTION

The majority of people with a developmental disorder (DD) function in the range of mild cognitive impairment (Friedlander et al. 2003; Waldman et al. 2006) and can be accommodated in a general practice with a little extra training, understanding, and effort. Treating patients with developmental disabilities in the dental office does not require a whole new set of skills but rather an adaptation of the ones already possessed by the provider (National Institute of Dental and Craniofacial Research 2009).

## PERSONAL INFORMATION

Ideally the initial patient interview/collection of personal information should be done over the phone prior to the first visit, but it could also be accomplished at the first appointment in a quiet and private space away from the distractions of a busy office. A "quiet room" if available may give the patient a chance to sit in the dental chair and become accustomed to the surroundings in a nonthreatening manner. You may also consider having only a single person, or perhaps two, be present during the interview to decrease the level of stimulation and allow the patient to become familiar with the provider and assistant.

*Treating the Dental Patient with a Developmental Disorder*, First Edition.
Edited by Karen A. Raposa and Steven P. Perlman.
© 2012 John Wiley & Sons, Inc. Published 2012 by John Wiley & Sons, Inc.

The majority of minor children with DD reside with their families and will most likely present with a parent as a primary caregiver. In that case collecting personal information such as address, phone number, parents' names, and emergency contact information should be routine. In addition, it is important to collect the contact information of the pediatrician (or primary care physician) as well as any specialists involved in the patient's care. You may also wish to collect other data that may be useful and relevant, such as where the patient attends school, type of class, and other therapies the patient may be receiving (i.e., occupational, physical, or speech therapy). Since you may wish at some point to contact other professionals involved in the patient's care, it is prudent to get the parent's permission to do so from the start.

While some adults with DD may live independently in the community, many reside with their families or in a community residence. For patients who reside on their own and are their own guardians, collecting the necessary information may take a bit more effort. It is important to remember that individuals with an intellectual disability will show deficits not only in cognitive functioning but also in adaptive functioning as well (National Institute of Dental and Craniofacial Research 2009).

Adaptive skills are functional life skills such as communication, self-care, and social interpersonal skills. Therefore, the practitioner should be prepared to assist the patient if necessary. The patient may have a social worker, case worker, friend, or family member who helps him or her with health care logistics/access and decisions. It is critical to identify if such a party exists as this person may be of great help in facilitating treatment. It is also key to be sure to obtain the patient's permission to share information with the third party in order not to violate any Health Insurance Portability and Accountability Act (HIPAA) regulations.

Other adult patients may reside in a community-based group residence and in this situation the dental practitioner may have little or no contact with a patient's family members (Romer & Filanova 2006). While this may appear problematic at first, in reality this may be one of the more easily navigated scenarios. Patients who live in such a setting usually will be accompanied by a direct care staff member (caregiver) who will have all the essential information in a binder or a "big book" that contains guardian information and records of past medical and dental visits, as well as behavioral and social information (Romer & Filanova 2006). The agency that runs the residence usually requires a consult form be filled out that documents the dental visit. A written request on this form is also a good way to obtain any other necessary information.

Of course, adults with DD may also live at home with their families. In this case, a parent or other family member will most likely be the resource for your basic information. It is important to note that even if an adult with DD lives with a parent, that parent may not be the legal guardian and may not be able to consent to treatment. It is imperative that a practitioner be familiar with the guardianship laws in the state in which he or she practices, as they vary quite a bit (Romer 2009).

# FAMILY DYNAMICS

Parents of children with disabilites report more stress than those of typically developing children (Boyd 2002). Such parents also report a feeling that providers do not actively listen to their concerns and may not respond in a supportive manner (Minnes & Steiner 2009). While it is always important to build a strong patient-provider bond, it is critical in this population. There are several issues that one needs to consider that are unique to this situation. These parents have suffered a loss of typical child ideation; that is, while they love the child with a disability, it is not what they expected. There is a wonderful poem by Emily Perl Kingsley, mother of a child with a developmental disability, entitled "Welcome to Holland." It likens the experience of having a child with a disability to planning a trip to Italy and ending up in Holland. There is loss and disappointment but also beauty and joy. Understanding that a parent may be overwhelmed with responsibilities such as other children, a spouse, a job, running a household, doctor/therapy appointments, and financial crises will help foster a bond. As a provider, you only have limited contact with this patient. A parent has that responsibility and stress 24 hours a day. Having a child who may have abberant behaviors and/or look different from other children can result in parents feeling isolated from other "typical" families. Other kinds of social isolation might include inability to attend church, work, or even go to a restaurant. These types of social and community interactions that we take for granted may not be a part of your patient's life. It is important to recognize that parents who have experienced this may be initially wary in any new setting, fearing rejection or discrimination. Also, it does not mitigate these issues just because that parent's child is now an adult. In fact, these feelings may be exacerbated by loss of other typical milestones such as a child going off to college, getting married, and having children of his or her own. (N.B. This is not to imply that these things are not possible for people with DD, but rather that the patients discussed here are adults who still require the supervision and caregiving of a parent and are less likely to achieve these milestones.) Setting the stage for a successful first visit is of paramount importance!

During the interview it is key to discuss who the primary caregiver is. It may be a parent, grandparent, sibling, other relative, or professional home health care assistant. Understanding who the patient lives with and who the primary caregiver is will give a better overview of the family dynamic.

This is also true for patients who reside in community-based residences. Important questions include: Who is the primary caregiver? Does this patient work better with a particular staff member? Have the residents of the home been together a long time? Does the patient have a roommate, someone he or she is close to? What are the "family" dynamics of the residence? How does the patient fit in with/get along with his or her housemates and staff?

Another aspect of patients' personal situations you may wish to delve into is about hobbies or things he/she like to do. What is their typical day like? What kinds of activities do he/she enjoy? Many practitioners use patients' interests to foster a bond, whether it is a favorite sport, hobby, television show, or other interest. Our patients with developmental disabilites are no different. Patients love to talk about themselves and share, so ask the patient or the caregiver what kinds of activities the patient enjoys and what things he or she likes to do.

Another suggestion is to explore a "day in the life"; that is, have the patient or caregiver describe a typical day to you. You may be surprised to find out that most patients are VERY busy!

## DENTAL EXPERIENCES

Taking a good history of dental experiences is especially important when providing care for patients with developmental disabilities. Some suggested questions might be: What is the patient's cognitive ability? How does the patient communicate (i.e., make his or her needs known if nonverbal)? How can the patient's behavior in a stressful situation be characterized? How has the patient reacted to previous dental treatment? How has dental treatment been accomplished in the past? Does the patient have any particular sensitivity such as air, water spray, fluorescent lighting, loud noises, reclined position (Meurs et al. 2010; Dougherty & MacRae 2006)? All of these questions will aid in your planning for successful treatment. If a patient has not had previous dental treatment, questions regarding reaction to medical examinations, vaccinations, blood draws, and so forth may also prove useful. However, while these may be similarly invasive, patients may react differently than predicted when it comes to the "invasion of the mouth."

Asking about the home care routine is also recommended. Questions such as: What kinds of problems have been encountered during home care? Does the patient cooperate? Who does the brushing? If the patient is a self-brusher, is the activity supervised? What kind of products does the patient use? Is flossing tolerated? Rinsing? Power/electric toothbrushing? Does the patient have a favorite flavor and/or brand of toothpaste? If the patient is a self-brusher, or uses minimal assistance, this may be a good time to have the patient show the provider how he or she brushes his or her teeth.

Finally, a discussion of caregiver/patient expectations should take place. What are hygiene goals? Treatment expectations? Can they be reasonably accomplished? Will they be in the best interest of the patient in your expert opinion? Can the expected/planned treatment be maintained?

## ORAL HABITS

Patients with DD may present with atypical oral habits, and it is important to ask questions regarding these practices during the interview. Is the patient a frequent snacker, perhaps trying to obtain oral sensory satisfaction thoughout the day with various foods? What kinds of snacks does the person eat? (Cariogenicity may play a role in the overall clinical picture.) Some patients may have food aversions or preferences based on texture, always choosing soft foods, or perhaps hard, crunchy items (Raposa 2009). Other people may have a preferred taste sensation such as salty or sweet. Research has shown a relationship between food refusal and negative social skills in people with DD (Matson et al. 2006). Asking about regular dietary intake may give the practitioner insight into a patient's preferences and habits.

Patients with DD, especially children, may be receiving speech or occupational therapy on a regular basis. Sometimes food is used during therapy to aid in a particular activity or movement, or simply as a reward. Parents and caregivers also may use food as a positive reinforcer for a job well done or an activity accomplished. In addition, food may be used to pacify a person who is acting out. The use of food as a reward should be strictly discouraged. You might suggest positive words of encouragement, nonfood rewards such as a small toy, or time enjoying a favorite activity (i.e., watching television, playing a game) as a good substitute for a high-calorie snack. Likewise the threat of removal of the desired object/activity can also be powerful. It is important to ask the primary caregiver which approach works best with the patient. Of course the reward, or removal of the reward, must be something valued by the patient, and it is important that the caregiver and the dental provider all be on the same page if this strategy is to be successfully employed during an office visit.

Another issue that should be raised is that of nonintuitive behaviors, especially ones that may result in self-injurious behavior (SIB). SIB is defined as committing intentional acts that result in tissue or organ damage (Pies & Popli 1995). These can range from seemingly innocuous acts such as nail biting, continuing along to bruxism, and all the way to skin cutting and auto-amputation. From that standpoint, sensory chewing, that is, chewing on nonfood items such as rubber tubing, washcloths, and so on, as well as bruxism can be considered SIB. Sensory chewing has been suggested by some to perhaps aid in the relief of stress or to provide stimulation to the masticatory muscles (Raposa 2009). Interestingly, patients with psychiatric disorders who are not intellectually impaired but engage in SIB have reported using it as a type of relief from psychic pain or tension

(Cordas et al. 2006; Herpertz 1995). It is not clear if such habits serve the same purpose in patients with DD, although for patients who are blind, eye poking is thought to be a self-stimulatory activity (Hyman et al. 1990). It has been speculated that SIB for people with DD is an escalation of stereotypies (purposeless repetitive movements) and may serve the same function; that is, to self-stimulate. Many patients will clench or grind habitually or in response to a stressor. Traditional dental therapies such as nightguards may be employed, but compliance may be an issue. Construction of more advanced appliances may be needed, including those with retentive clasps, permanently cemented appliances, or even fixed prosthodontics.

Other atypical oral habits that may be present are pica (the ingestion of nonfood items) and mouthing of nonfood objects (toys, clothes, etc.). Pica can result in severe intestinal damage as well as poisoning (McAdam et al. 2004) Patients may ingest dirt, pencils, paint chips, or any number of harmful items. Toothpaste is quite often on this list and parents may feel it is something of less concern, as it belongs in the mouth. However, it is important to know if the patient exhibits this behavior and help caregivers understand the risks and develop a plan to keep such items out of reach. Of course, patients may simply have a thumb- or finger-sucking habit and this may present its own challenges. The pediatric dental and orthodontic literature abounds with information regarding habit-breaking treatments, but realize that in a patient with DD, it may be even more difficult. People with DD often have concomitant medical conditions, and some of these may require a special diet (National Institute of Dental and Craniofacial Research 2009). For example, there are reports of a higher incidence of celiac disease in people with some types of DD (Percy & Propst 2008) and this is noteworthy, as these patients are on a strict gluten-free diet. There has been speculation and anecdotal reports that a gluten-free diet may be of benefit for people with DD who do not have documented celiac disease. However, the current scientific evidence does not support this theory. That is not to say this may not be of some benefit, but rather that the evidence to support this as a therapy does not currently exist. The most common comorbidity found in patients with DD is epilepsy. (Robbins 2009) Since the 1920s, physicians have been using a ketogenic diet for patients with drug-resistant epilepsy (Neal 2008). This high-fat, restricted-carbohydrate diet mimics starvation and results in the body using ketone bodies to meet the basic fuel demands of brain and body function (Hartman et al. 2007). While the exact mechanism of action of this diet is still unclear, it has been shown in several studies to be effective in children with epilepsy who have a history of intractible seizures (Freeman et al. 1998; Kang et al. 2005; Coppola et al. 2002; Kankirawatana et al. 2001; Maydell et al. 2001; Vining et al. 1998). Such specialized diets are not without side effects, and patients may be at risk for clinical nutrient deficiency (Kirby & Danner 2009). Providers should familiarize themselves with any specialized diet a patient may be on and be sure to look for possible oral side effects of nutritional deficiencies.

## BEHAVIOR/EMOTIONS

A behavior history and information about a person's specific needs can aid in delivering more person-centered, individualized care in the least stresssful setting for all parties involved (Meurs et al. 2010).

Unfortunately, most oral health providers have not had training in taking a behavioral history with the possible exception of pediatric dentists. For patients with DD a behavioral history is very important (Romer & Filanova 2006). Some patients with DD may react with fear at a new place, provider, and experience (National Institute of Dental and Craniofacial Research 2009). Consultation with a parent, caregiver, guardian, or direct care staff regarding the patient's past behavior can be invaluable in avoiding pitfalls and can be the key to treatment success. Asking questions regarding impulsivity and how a patient behaves when frustrated or angry is a good place to start. You may also wish to use a standardized form that has a comprehensive list of questions such as: Does the patient use avoidance to get out of unpleasant tasks, that is, frequent requests to use the restroom or inappropriate anti-social behavior? Is the patient combative or aggressive? Is the patient self-injurious? (If the patient has had episodes of self-injurious behavior or is currently exhibiting such behavior, more information may be needed.) Is this behavior being used for avoidance or another purpose? The head and neck are the most common areas of SIB. However, this does not mean the patient has pain of dental origin. SIB is an involved behavior and may be an indication that the individual needs referral to a specialty center for care. Treatment may be beyond the scope of the novice to the practice of dentistry for people with DD (Romer & Dougherty 2009). Does the patient have vocal outbursts? What stimulates these types of behaviors? What approaches work best with this patient? How does this patient learn best? Is this patient a visual or auditory learner? What calms the patient? Does music help? How does the patient respond to music? If the patient loses control, how can it be regained? Does the patient respond to voice commands? Are there other behavioral strategies that work better to calm the patient and regain control? What types of reinforcers are successful? Maybe most importantly, what DOESN'T work with this person?

Two easy-to-use forms that can facilitate a behavioral history are available from the New York State Office for People with Developmental Disabilities (http://www.opwdd.ny.gov/opwdd_services_supports/oral_health/forms), one a long, very comprehensive four-page form and the other a shorter form. From a practical standpoint, it is ideal to have this form filled out by a parent or guardian ahead of time and then have it available for review at the appointment.

Finally, it is important to remember that patients with DD and their families want what other patients want: to be treated with respect and compassion in a professional and caring environment.

# REFERENCES

Boyd BA. (2002). Examining the relationship between stress and lack of social support in mothers of children with autism. *Focus on Autism and Other Developmental Disabilities* 17:208–215.

Coppola G, Veggiotti P, Cusmai R, et al. (2002). The ketogenic diet in children, adolescents and young adults with refractory epilepsy: An Italian multicentric experience. *Epilepsy Research* 48(3):221–227.

Cordas TA, et al. (2006). Oxcarbezepine for self-mutilating bulimic patients. *International Journal of Neuropsychopharmacology* 9:769–771.

Dougherty N, MacRae R. (2006). Providing dental care to patients with developmental disabilities: An introduction for the private practitioner. *New York State Dental Journal* 72(2):29–32.

Freeman JM, Vining EP, Pillas DJ, et al. (1998). The efficacy of the ketogenic diet. *Pediatrics* 102:1358–1363.

Friedlander AH, Yagiela JA, Paterno VI, et al. (2003). The pathophysiology, medical management and dental implications of Fragile X, Rett and Prader-Willi syndromes. *California Dental Journal* 31(9):693–702.

Hartman AL, Gasior M, Vining EP, et al. (2007). The neuropharmacology of the ketogenic diet. *Pediatric Neurology* 36:281–292.

Herpertz S. (1995). Self-injurious behavior: Psychopathological and nosological characteristics in subtypes of self-injurers. *Acta Psychiatrica Scandinavia* 91:57–68.

Hyman S, Fisher W, Mercugliano M, et al. (1990). Children with self-injurious behavior. *Pediatrics* 85:437–441.

Kang HC, Kim YJ, Kim DW, et al. (2005). Efficacy and safety of the ketogenic diet for intractable childhood epilepsy: Korean multicentric experience. *Epilepsia* 46(2):272–279.

Kankirawatana P, Jirapinyo P, Kankirawatana S, et al. (2001). Ketogenic diet: An alternative treatment for refractory epilepsy in children. *Journal of the Medical Association of Thailand* 84(7):1027–1032.

Kirby M, Danner E. (2009). Nutritional deficiencies in children on restricted diets. *Pediatric Clinics of North America* 56:1085–1103.

Matson JL, Cooper CL, Mayville SB, et al. (2006). The relationship between food refusal and social skills in persons with intellectual disabilities. *Journal of Intellectual and Developmental Disability* 31(1):47–52.

Maydell BV, Wyllie E, Akhtar N, et al. (2001). Efficacy of the ketogenic diet in focal versus generalized seizures. *Pediatric Neurology* 25:208–212.

McAdam DB, Sherman JA, Sheldon JB, et al. (2004). Behavioral interventions to reduce the pica of persons with developmental disabilities. *Behavior Modification* 28(1):45–72.

Meurs D, Rutten M, Jongh A. (2010). Does information about patients who are intellectually disabled translate into better cooperation during dental visits? *Special Care Dentistry* 30(5):200–205.

Minnes P, Steiner K. (2009). Parent's views on enhancing the quality of health care for their children with fragile X syndrome, autism or Down syndrome. *Child: Care, Health and Development* 35(2):250–256.

National Institute of Dental and Craniofacial Research. (2009). Practical oral care for people with developmental disabilities. NIH Publication No. 09-5196.

Neal EG, Chaffe H, Schwartz RH, et al. (2008). The ketogenic diet for the treatment of childhood epilepsy: A randomised controlled trial. *Lancet Journal* 7:500–506.

Percy M, Propst E. (2008). Celiac disease: Its many faces and relevance to developmental disabilities. *Journal on Developmental Disabilities* 14(2):105–110.

Pies R, Popli A. (1995). Self-injurious behavior: Pathophysiology and implications for treatment. *Journal of Clinical Psychiatry* 56(12):580–588.

Raposa KA. (2009). Behavioral management for patients with intellectual and developmental disorders. *Dental Clinics of North America: The Special Care Patient* 53(2):359–373.

Robbins MR. (2009). Dental management of special needs patients who have epilepsy. *Dental Clinics of North America: The Special Care Patient* 53(2):295–309.

Romer M. (2009). Consent, restraint and people with special needs: A review. *Special Care in Dentistry* 29(1):58–66.

Romer M, Dougherty N. (2009). Oral self-injurious behaviors in patients with developmental disabilities. *Dental Clinics of North America: The Special Care Patient* 53(2):339–350.

Romer M, Filanova V. (2006). Providing dental care to patinents with developmental disabilities: Medical/legal issues. *New York State Dental Journal* 72(2):36–37.

Vining EP, Freeman JM, Ballaban-Gil K, et al. (1998). A multicenter study of the efficacy of the ketogenic diet. *Archives of Neurology* 55:1433–1437.

Waldman HB, Truhlar MR, Perlman SP. (2006). Slipping through the cracks: Dental care for older persons with intellectual disabilities. *New York State Dental Journal* 72(2):47–51.

# Medical/developmental review/ interview

## Martha Ann Keels, DDS, PhD

In order to provide safe, effective, and compassionate care for patients with a developmental disorder (DD), one must carefully ascertain their medical history (Balzer 2007; Crall 2007; Dougherty & MacRae 2006).

Whether a paper charting system or an electronic health record is used, one must ensure that the content of the medical questionnaire is comprehensive and addresses a potentially complex medical history. A separate surgical history form may be indicated to help the parent/caregiver record this data. Having the parent/caregiver complete the medical history prior to the appointment is time saving. Also having access to the patient's electronic medical health record is ideal. This allows the dentist to validate the information given as well as to ensure critical information was not overlooked. Having the staff who schedule the appointments determine if a new patient has a specific diagnosis (i.e., Hurler's syndrome, Rett syndrome) is very helpful, as it affords the dentist adequate time to review any materials regarding that condition prior to meeting the patient. Prior review of the medical history by the dentist will allow sufficient time to then educate the dental staff on any special precautions that should be taken with the patient. Useful websites to access information on developmental disorders include PubMed and OMIM (Online Mendelian Inheritance in Man).

It is important to collect a complete medical history in order to guide one's decision on how to best clinically examine the patient with a developmental disorder. Sometimes it is best to leave the patient in their wheelchair

*Treating the Dental Patient with a Developmental Disorder*, First Edition.
Edited by Karen A. Raposa and Steven P. Perlman.
© 2012 John Wiley & Sons, Inc. Published 2012 by John Wiley & Sons, Inc.

or sitting on the clinic floor, wherever the patient is most comfortable, while the parent/caregiver is being interviewed. This allows the parent to focus on the discussion with the dentist. The medical history will also guide one's treatment planning decisions on the urgency and extensiveness of dental care needed given the patient's quality of life and expected longevity (Glassman & Subar 2009). Decisions regarding whether to treat the patient in an outpatient clinic setting or in a hospital setting as well as the need for protective stabilization, sedation, or general anesthesia will also be influenced by the information obtained from the medical history (Waldman et al. 2009). This chapter will highlight areas of the medical history that may be unique to a patient with a developmental disorder.

## MEDICAL INFORMATION

The medical history form should enable the dentist to easily ascertain the overall diagnosis and any secondary conditions. Examples may be the child has Down syndrome and secondary conditions of an atrial septal heart defect and autism; a child with cerebral palsy and secondary conditions of a seizure disorder and gastroesophageal reflux; a child with spina bifida and secondary conditions of a latex allergy and a chiari malformation. Table 3.1 provides a comprehensive outline to guide the intake of a medical history. Table 3.2 contains a list of the medical conditions that should be listed in a medical history intake form for a patient with DD (AAPD 2010–2011). Table 3.3 provides a list of common DDs with their potential comorbidities. Patients with DD frequently have had

**Table 3.1**  Medical history intake outline (adapted from AAPD 2011/2012).

Name and nickname
Date of birth
Gender
Race/ethnicity
Height/weight their by report
Name, address, and telephone number of all physicians
Date of last physical examination
Immunization status
Summary of health problems
Any health conditions that necessitate antibiotics prior to dental treatment
Allergies/sensitivities/reactions to any medication, latex, food, dyes, metal, acrylic, or tapes
Current medications (including over-the-counter analgesics, vitamins, and herbal supplements). Document dose and frequency
Hospitalizations—reason, date, outcome
Surgeries—reason, date, outcome
Significant injuries—description, date, outcome

**Table 3.2**   Outline of medical conditions.

General:
  Complications during pregnancy and/or birth
  Prematurity
  Congenital anomalies
  Cleft lip/palate
  Inherited disorders
  Nutritional deficiencies
  Problems of growth or stature

Head, ears, eyes, nose, and throat:
  Lesions in/around mouth
  Chronic adenoid/tonsil infections
  Chronic otitis media
  Ear problems
  Hearing impairments
  Eye problems
  Visual impairments
  Sinusitis
  Speech impairments
  Apnea/snoring
  Mouth breathing

Cardiovascular:
  Congenital heart defects/disease
  Heart murmur
  High blood pressure
  Rheumatic fever
  Rheumatic heart disease

Respiratory:
  Asthma
  Tuberculosis
  Cystic fibrosis
  Frequent colds/coughs
  Respiratory syncytial virus
  Reactive airway disease/breathing problems
  Smoking

Gastrointestinal:
  Eating disorder
  Ulcer
  Excessive gagging
  Gastroesophageal/acid reflux disease
  Hepatitis
  Jaundice
  Liver disease
  Intestinal problems
  Prolonged diarrhea
  Unintentional weight loss

(*Continued*)

**Table 3.2** *(cont'd)*.

Celiac disease
Lactose intolerance
Dietary restrictions

Genitourinary:
  Bladder infections
  Kidney infections
  Pregnancy
  Systemic birth control
  Sexually transmitted diseases

Musculoskeletal:
  Arthritis
  Scoliosis
  Bone/joint problems
  TMJ problems

Integumentary:
  Fever blisters
  Eczema
  Rash/hives
  Dermatologic conditions

Neurologic:
  Fainting
  Dizziness
  Autism
  Developmental disorders
  Learning problems/delays
  Mental disability
  Brain injury
  Cerebral palsy
  Seizures/convulsions
  Epilepsy
  Headaches/migraines
  Hydrocephaly
  Shunts—ventriculoperitoneal, ventriculoatrial, ventriculovenous

Psychiatric:
  Abuse
  Alcohol and chemical dependency
  Emotional disturbance
  Hyperactivity/attention deficit hyperactivity disorder

Endocrine:
  Diabetes
  Growth delays
  Hormonal problems
  Precocious puberty
  Thyroid problems

**Table 3.2**  (cont'd)

Hematologic/lymphatic/immunologic:
  Anemia
  Blood disorder
  Transfusion
  Excessive bleeding
  Bruising easily
  Hemophilia
  Sickle cell disease/trait
  Cancer, tumor, other malignancy
  Immune disorder
  Chemotherapy
  Radiation therapy
  Hematopoietic cell transplant

Infectious disease:
  Measles
  Mumps
  Rubella
  Scarlet fever
  Varicella (chicken pox)
  Mononucleosis
  Cytomegalovirus (CMV)
  Pertussis (whooping cough)
  Human immunodeficiency virus/acquired immune deficiency syndrome
  (HIV/AIDS)

Family history:
  Genetic disorders
  Problems with general anesthesia
  Serious medical conditions or illnesses

Social concerns:
  Passive smoke exposure
  Religious or philosophical objections to treatment

multiple surgeries. Therefore, providing the parents or caregivers with a form that allows them to list these surgical procedures is helpful. Table 3.4 contains a sample surgical history. The documented medical history will guide the dentist in the direction of important verbal questioning. An example of this would be noting the patient has whiplash shaken infant syndrome and then following up with questions regarding the child's aspiration risk and ability to see and inquiring if the child has an oral facial aversion.

In addition to ascertaining the medical diagnoses, it is important to assess the patient's developmental age in comparison to his or her chronological age. Being cognizant of the patient's developmental age is important in directing communication and behavior management techniques (Meurs et al. 2010).

**Table 3.3**   Examples of common comorbidities with developmental disorders.

| Primary diagnosis | Secondary medical conditions | | | |
|---|---|---|---|---|
| Autism spectrum disorders | Fragile X syndrome | Tuberous sclerosis | Seizure disorder | Tourette syndrome |
| Down syndrome | ASD, VSD | Autism | ALL (leukemia) | |
| Cerebral palsy | Seizure disorder | GERD (reflux) | G-tube fed | |
| Spina bifida | Latex sensitivity | Chiari malformation | Hydrocephaly | VP shunt |
| Celiac disease | Gluten sensitivity | Mouth ulcerations | | |
| Lesch-Nyhan syndrome | Oral Self-abuse | Cerebral palsy | Seizure disorder | |
| Whiplash shaken infant syndrome | Blind | Seizure disorder | Cerebral palsy | |
| Turner syndrome | Short stature | Coarctation of aorta | Kidney malformation | Hypothyroidism |
| Prader Willi syndrome | Obesity | Hypotonia | Hypogonadism | |

**Table 3.4**   Sample surgical history.

| Month/Year | Surgical procedure | Surgeon | Hospital | Notes |
|---|---|---|---|---|
| 9/2010 | Nissen fundoplication | Dr. Rice | General Hospital | No complications |
| 3/2011 | Gastrostomy tube placement | Dr. Rice | General Hospital | No Complications |
| 6/2011 | Hamstring release | Dr. Fitch | General Hospital | No Complications |

## MEDICATIONS/ALLERGIES/ANAPHYLAXIS RISK

Prior to examining a child with a DD, one must ensure that all of the potential risks that may affect the success of the patient's clinical evaluation and any subsequent treatment have been covered. Children with DD may have been exposed to more medications than other children, thereby increasing their chances of a documented allergic reaction or in an extreme case anaphylaxis. Documenting any drug reactions is important to alleviate the potential for anaphylaxis in the dental office. Children with DD may have also had more treatments involving urethral catheterization, enhancing their risk for a latex allergy; therefore the examining area will need to be free of all latex-containing items, such as rubber gloves, rubber dams and latex prophy cups. If the child has a sensitivity to gluten or celiac disease, then products with gluten such as certain prophy pastes should not be used (Percy & Propst 2008).

The need for an antibiotic premedication is also possible if the child has a cardiac defect requiring infective endocarditis prophylaxis, an indwelling venous catheter, or an impaired immune system whereby the neutrophil count is low. Consultation with the patient's physician is prudent to verify the need for antibiotic premedication. Published guidelines exist to guide the proper selection of antibiotic and dosage (AAPD 2011/2012).

## ASPIRATION RISK

The risk of aspiration is high among children with severe DD, as their gag reflex may be impaired and they may be too weak to cough independently. Identifying this risk is important to guide the dentist in positioning the patient for examination. If the child is in a wheelchair, then it may be prudent to complete the examination with the child in the wheelchair maintaining his or her normal upright position. If the child is able to be transferred to the dental chair, then positioning the dental chair in a more upright inclination may enhance keeping the airway open. If the child has an NPO status, then one should avoid saturating the oral cavity with water during any dental evaluations or treatment. If water is needed, then a moistened gauze may be used. Antibiotic prophylaxis may be indicated to prevent aspiration pneumonia, if aspiration of saliva or calculus is anticipated. If significant dental care is needed, then treatment in the operating room may be appropriate so that the airway can be protected with a throat pack.

## PARALYSIS RISK

If a child has a chiari malformation or an atlanto-axis instability, then the dentist must be vigilant about supporting the head and neck to avoid damage to the spinal cord and potential paralysis. Children with Down syndrome and Hurler's syndrome have an increased risk for head and neck instability. If the patient appears combative or agitated with a history of head and neck instability, then evaluation and dental cleaning under general anesthesia may be indicated.

## BONE FRACTURE RISK

Recognizing the risk of bone fracture prior to any evaluation is important. It may be in the patient's best interest to keep him or her in a wheelchair rather than risk dropping the patient during a transfer to the dental chair.

Patients with severe obesity may be best examined in their wheelchair. Conditions leading to fragile bones, such as osteoporosis or osteogenesis imperfecta, should alert the dentist to be very careful in handling the patient. Caregivers are usually excellent resources in how to best physically handle their child.

# SELF-INJURIOUS BEHAVIORS

In rarer situations, some children with DD have self-injurious behaviors. They may present to the dental office secured in such a way that they are not capable of any self-injurious behavior; the dentist should recognize this risk and maintain the same positioning and restraints to avoid any self-injury by the patient. Children with Lesch-Nyhan syndrome, congenital indifference to pain, or closed head injury have self-injurious behaviors (Hyman et al. 1990; Romer & Dougherty 2009). Table 3.5 summarizes the potential risks that need to be identified and managed carefully to ensure successful care of the patient with DD.

# SENSORY CONCERNS

There are other concerns that need to be identified to ensure a successful patient encounter. These concerns are not life threatening or as potentially medically complicating as the risks identified in Table 3.6, but they are important to recognize in order to communicate effectively with the patient as well as make the examination as comfortable as possible. After the medical diagnosis and comorbidities history have been reviewed and the developmental age documented, then the dentist should inquire about the patient's sensory awareness, in particular vision, hearing, smelling, and touch (Table 3.6) (Raposa 2009).

Inquiring about the child's visual acuity is important to avoid startling the patient as well as to guide the language used by the dentist and staff. It would be inappropriate to ask the patient if he or she would like to watch the dental procedure in the mirror if the patient cannot see. Welcoming a see and eye dog (also called seeing eye dog) into the clinic would be appropriate for a patient accustomed to being escorted by a guide dog. Honoring the see and eye dog rules is also important, as one must ask permission to pet a see and eye dog. Do not be offended if the owner says no, as in many cases when the dog is working no petting is allowed. Recognizing light sensitivity is also important. A patient with sensitivity to light should be offered sunglasses to wear while the examining light is being used. Selecting an examination room without windows or closing blinds in the room may also comfort a patient with light sensitivity. The

**Table 3.5**  Summary of potential risks that need to be ascertained prior to performing the dental exam on a patient with DD.

Allergic reaction/anaphylaxis
Infection risk
NPO status and aspiration risk
Paralysis risk
Bone fracture risk
Self-injury risk
Provider-injury risk (biting, hitting, pinching)

**Table 3.6**  Potential sensory concerns that affect examining the patient with DD.

Visual impairment—light sensitivity, blindness
Hearing impairment—noise sensitivity, deafness
Taste and smell sensitivity
Touch sensitivity—oral facial aversion

dentist must also be sensitive to patients with one functioning eye or limited peripheral vision and make certain to engage within the patient's visual field.

Identifying patients with any noise sensitivity, such as covering ears to the sound of a vacuum cleaner or a train, is important to avoid a startle reaction to the prophy or the handpieces. Having earplugs or noise-cancelling headphones is a helpful aid to making noise-sensitive patients more comfortable. Recognizing a patient with deafness is also important. If one ear is better than another, then one would talk toward the ear with better hearing. If one can hear if the volume is increased, then the dentist should also talk louder in order to be heard by the patient. If the deafness is severe, then the dentist may have to use sign language or arrange for an interpreter familiar with sign language skills.

Taste and smell sensitivities are also important to identify, as the dentist can minimize the exposure to certain tastes as well as reduce any potential odors that may trigger an adverse response. If the child has oral facial aversion, then the severity of the condition will have to be determined in order to select the most appropriate behavior guidance technique (i.e., desensitization, general anesthesia). Recognizing the sensory concerns of the patient will enhance the success of the dental care. Having a system whereby you earmark the patient's health record with an alert that reminds you of the patient's sensory concerns helps ensure excellent patient care.

Given the complexity of the patient's medical history, the dentist may need to spend the allotted appointment time reviewing the medical and dental history, leaving the dental clinical examination and any treatment needs (cleaning, extractions, etc.) to a subsequent appointment.

# REFERENCES

American Academy of Pediatric Dentistry. (2011/2012). Guideline on record-keeping. *Pediatric Dentistry* 33(special issue):277–284.

———. (2011/2012). Management of dental patients with special health care needs. *Pediatric Dentistry* 33(special issue):142–146.

———. (2011/2012). *2011/2012 AAPD Reference Manual*. Chicago: AAPD.

Balzer J. (2007). Improving systems of care for people with special needs: The ASTDD Best Practices Project. *Pediatric Dentistry* 29(2):123–128.

Crall J. (2007). Improving oral health for individuals with special health care needs. *Pediatric Dentistry* 29(2):98–104.

Dougherty N, MacRae R. (2006). Providing dental care to patients with developmental disabilities: An introduction for the private practitioner. *New York State Dental Journal* 72(2):29–32.

Glassman P, Subar P. (2009). Planning dental treatment for people with special needs. *Dental Clinics of North America: The Special Care Patient* 53(2):195–206.

Hyman S, Fisher W, Mercugliano M, et al. (1990). Children with self-injurious behavior. *Pediatrics* 85:437–441.

Meurs D, Rutten M, Jongh A. (2010). Does information about patients who are intellectually disabled translate into better cooperation during dental visits? *Special Care Dentistry* 30(5):200–205.

Percy M, Propst E. (2008). Celiac disease: Its many faces and relevance to developmental disabilities. *Journal on Developmental Disabilities* 14(2):105–110.

Raposa KA. (2009). Behavioral management for patients with intellectual and developmental disorders. *Dental Clinics of North America: The Special Care Patient* 53(2):359–373.

Romer M, Dougherty N. (2009). Oral self-injurious behaviors in patients with developmental disabilities. *Dental Clinics of North America: The Special Care Patient* 53(2):339–350.

Waldman HB, Rader R, Perlman SP. (2009). Health related issues for individuals with special health care needs. *Dental Clinics of North America: The Special Care Patient* 53(2):183–194.

# Treatment considerations

## Section 1: Behavioral supports

Ray A. Lyons, DDS, FADPD, DABSCD

*Dental education typically teaches students to perform procedures on "well" (healthy) patients and "well-behaved" patients.*

*Human behavior is sculpted by discipline, rules, boundaries, structure, and applied social pressures and is best learned when factors are consistently applied by a respected source.*

*General anesthesia should not be the immediate treatment of choice for tantrum, maladaptive, or noncompliant behavior, or for the person with developmental disorders.*

*The potential for building a trusted relationship, and treatment success, will be determined by a dental team's shared philosophy and dedicated approach to behavioral support.*

## INTRODUCTION

Patients with developmental disorders often present a challenge for the dental care team. The exacting and surgical nature of dental procedures requires significant patient cooperation to ensure safe delivery of care; yet the discipline of special care dentistry is charged to provide comprehensive care to patients with a complex variety of cooperative, cognitive, and physical abilities in the least restrictive manner (Fenton et al. 1987). In due course, the effective practitioner, as teacher, must dynamically work to

*Treating the Dental Patient with a Developmental Disorder*, First Edition.
Edited by Karen A. Raposa and Steven P. Perlman.
© 2012 John Wiley & Sons, Inc. Published 2012 by John Wiley & Sons, Inc.

support the patient with developmental disorders in a fashion that builds the patient's coping behavior and helps him or her participate in meaningful clinical treatment.

There is a perceived hierarchy of methodology available to dentistry to assist patients in their attempt to cope with clinical oral health treatment (ADA 2007; AAPD 2006b). These techniques range from tell-show-do, to medical stabilization, to general anesthesia. This chapter intends to review the principles of basic behavioral support as the fundamental starting point of this hierarchy and to examine how those principles apply to assisting people with developmental disorders during clinical care using the least restrictive approach. The practitioner who successfully facilitates patient cooperation without resorting to use of advanced techniques (pharmacologic, medical stabilization, general anesthesia) theoretically opens a door for patient access to comprehensive oral care in a traditional setting for a lifetime.

## INTERDISCIPLINARY COMPARISON: DENTISTRY'S UNIQUE TASK

Most people with developmental disorders must utilize some or all of the following entities within the health care system: primary and specialty physician care, routine nursing supervision, pharmacological management, a full spectrum of therapy support services (occupational, physical, speech and language, behavioral, dietary, etc.), case management, and/or assistance with skills of daily living. Although this segment of our population often poses a unique challenge to all in health care, few disciplines face the extremely delicate and exigent task required of dentistry. "*Clinical dental treatment is the most exacting and demanding medical procedure that persons with developmental disorders undergo on a regular basis throughout their lifetime. Dental treatment is basically surgical in nature, usually requiring controlled placement of sharpened instrumentation in intimate proximity to the face, airway, and highly vascularized and innervated oral tissues*" (Lyons 2004). Thus, impulsive patient movements during a *dental debridement* easily pose as much of a threat of serious injury, as the same movements during a true *surgical procedure*.

Most dentists would claim that clinical treatment is challenging enough with a cooperative patient. It is no wonder that many practitioners perceive that advanced behavioral support/management modalities, such as sedation and general anesthesia, are necessary to safely treat many people with developmental disorders. Certainly, most medical surgeons wouldn't proceed without such control. Yet by utilizing noninvasive, nonpharmacological behavioral support techniques, philosophies, and combined approaches, many dentists are able to provide meaningful care in moderately routine fashion to many people with developmental disorders, without resorting to use of deep sedation or general anesthesia.

# AN UNDENIABLE CHALLENGE: BEHAVIORAL SUPPORT AS A BARRIER TO ACCESS

*When my patient is "all stressed out", I have a hard time not getting "all stressed out" myself!*

Dental team member

*Clapping for our patient upon completion of care can actually serve as a celebration (and an emotional release) for all: "that was tough,* but we all did it!*"*

Special care team member

With the possible exception of many readers of this book, a *majority of dentists* have doubts regarding their own skill or feel inadequately trained in patient behavioral support, especially when it is applied to people with developmental disorders (Casamassimo et al. 2004). Clevenger et al. (1993) found that 80% of dentists surveyed were unwilling to treat patients with developmental disabilities because of their resistive behavior. To place this evidence in perspective, Casamassimo et al. (2004) showed that patient behavior was almost 3 times more likely to be named as a high-level barrier to care than *lack of funds*.

This is not surprising if one considers that a study by Romer et al. (1999) documented the fact that most dental students received little didactic, clinical, and hands-on training in care of persons with disabilities). And Casamassimo et al. (2004) found that 40% of practicing dentists described additional training pertinent to treatment of people with developmental disorders to be desirable or very desirable. Although some dental educators have renewed an emphasis on training students in special needs care (Thierer & Meyerowitz 2005), current evidence still suggests that most dental students fail to receive adequate experience in mediating patient behavior related to dental treatment.

One reason dentists consider behavioral support to be one of the most challenging aspects of care of persons with developmental disorders is that studies identify that a patient's behavioral stress and anxiety are reflected and transmitted to the members of the dental team (Feigal 2001; Reese & Alexander 2002; Do 2004). Burtner and Dicks (1994) found that private practitioners tend to avoid patients with developmental disorders and react with frustration or apathy related to the maladaptive behaviors they exhibit. In another study, one-third of dentists actually reported personally *feeling aggression* toward their physically resistive patients (Peretz et al. 2003). On occasion, physical resistance can escalate to the point of property damage or physical aggression toward caregivers and dental personnel (Waldman & Perlman 1997). Additionally, the patient who behaviorally resists treatment creates an ethical and legal burden for the practitioner (Griffen & Schneiderman 1992).

To further understand the barrier, Casamassimo states that unlike physicians, "adult-oriented general practices have little interest in or ability (time and skill) to manage parental/family issues" that are commonly inherent in the behavioral care of both children and adults with developmental disorders (Feigal 2001; Casamassimo 2006). Moreover, reimbursement seldom compensates a practice for the extra time and effort that is often needed to behaviorally support people with complex developmental disorders (Glassman et al. 2005).

In conclusion and before we get too deeply into this chapter's discussion of behavioral support for our *patients*, it may be wise to consider the fact that *dental professionals* need to reflect upon/develop their own mechanisms of support in working with this special population. The healthy dental team must construct strategies that mediate the personal stress inherent in challenging patient care. Examples might include pretreatment staff "huddles" to discuss anticipated behavioral approach/response, rest periods for the staff (as well as for the patient), posttreatment staff discussions, mutual compliments for team efforts, and even appropriate humor to lighten the mood (we are all human, after all). The team should focus on the fact that patient's skills are progressively learned and, traditionally, "*it gets better with time.*" Care of the person with developmental disorders involves so much more than just the procedure. Thus, the ultimate reward of behavioral support may be development of patient/practitioner relationships that define the essence of "health caring." Some of our most challenging patients will ultimately become our most gratifying success stories!

## BEHAVIORAL SUPPORT: "NO ONE LIKES TO BE *MANAGED*"

"Behavior management" has been the traditional term that describes the effort by families, caregivers, therapists, and also dentists to *control* disruptive behaviors of people with developmental disorders during daily activities or clinical treatment. Advocates have tried to help others understand that "no one likes to be managed" and that such terminology somewhat stigmatizes or dehumanizes the individual. Through life experience, every human grows, learns, and benefits from many sources of support and guidance in order to function in social and family settings. Thus, the American Academy of Pediatric Dentistry (AAPD) has changed its terminology from "behavior management" to "behavioral guidance" to better describe a continuum of individualized interaction involving the dentist and patient directed toward communication and education "which ultimately builds trust and allays fear and anxiety" (AAPD 2006b). In a synonymous and complementary fashion, the term "behavioral support" is used to describe a collaborative philosophy that is person-centered in that it considers the individual, evaluates his or her environment and support resources, and attempts to plan how challenging behavior can best be moderated (Governor's Commission on Mental

Retardation 1994). Families, care staff, and health care providers assume the role of teacher in the effort to assist people with developmental disorders gain skills that allow them to participate in activities, adapt to stressful situations, and tolerate medical treatment in as typical a manner as possible.

Several authors suggest that the majority of people with developmental disorders can receive routine dental care in the conventional dental office, presenting minimal or no behavior management difficulties for the dentist (Fenton et al. 1987; Subarian 2001: SAID 2001a). However, there are still many people with developmental disorders who present with unique and complex characteristics that challenge the dental practitioner's traditional approach to care. There are those people with developmental disorders who are affected with cognitive or physical impairments that complicate basic communication with the dental team (Yellowitz et al. 2004; AAPD 2006a). Other people with developmental disorders present with repetitive behaviors, psychiatric symptoms, and even aggression that may disrupt care (Friedlander et al. 2003). Uncontrolled, impulsive, or intentional body movements may endanger patient safety and pose a risk of injury to dental staff (SAID 2001b). Patients who demonstrate short attention spans may complicate the control needed for complex treatment. And many patients with developmental disorders may lack a "cognizance of benefit to cooperate," as they may be unable to appreciate the risks or consequences of their own actions, including refusal of care. Finally, studies have shown that people with developmental disorders have a greater level of fear and anxiety to seeking dental treatment than the general population (Gordon et al. 1998). If the dental team is not familiar with strategies for successfully accommodating the behavior of patients with developmental disorders, the tendency is to refuse to treat the person and refer him or her *somewhere else*. Depending on the community or region, that *"somewhere else"* may be hours away, may be overwhelmed by treatment demands, or may not exist at all.

## THE PATIENT AS A PERSON: "GET TO KNOW ME"

*More alike than different.*

National Down Syndrome Congress

*If you've met one person with autism, you've met one person with autism.*

Common saying in the autism field

*You treat my son like he's a real person!*

a mother participating in complex, disruptive, and demanding clinical dental treatment

*Stigmatization*—we see a wheelchair as the defining characteristic of the person using it.

We easily recognize dentistry's challenge, but the practitioner must also understand the multifaceted challenge faced by the patient. A person with developmental disorders must be granted the respect and dignity that we extend to any patient. Much of the etiology of "disability behavior" may simply be reflective of basic human needs, human coping mechanisms, and/or attempts to communicate, and should serve as a reminder that each of us shares similar attributes central to our humanity. People with developmental disorders share our common desires for safety, comfort, and attention, and experience anxiety and uncertainty, just as we might when we face situations that are unfamiliar to us. We should respectfully understand that these patients' lives may be complicated by limitations in problem-solving skills, coping skills, cognitive processes, motor abilities, psychological assets, developmental experience, and balanced sensory input (Sundheim & Ryan 1999). Thus as we reflect on our own daily challenges, it should be easy to understand anxiety and frustration in their lives.

One of the starting points of behavioral support for persons with developmental disorders is the dental team's discovery of patients' unique and varied personalities. They can be affectionate and sharing while being exceedingly stubborn. They may also be exceedingly frank and honest, so be careful not to ask a question you don't want to know the answer to! Some may be mischievous and it is delightful to discover those who possess a wicked sense of humor. But each as an individual will have strengths and weaknesses. Persons with developmental disorders almost never ask you to feel sorry for them; they simply ask that you make the effort to get to know them.

## EXPECTATIONS, FEAR, AND LEARNING TO COPE

*You won't be able to do anything with her.*
A mother's statement at the time of the initial appointment

*I did it, I did it!*
A 26-year-old man's exclamation to his mother as he returns to the waiting area upon completion of his first restoration

A basic conceptualization assumes that people with developmental disorders possess the ability to learn (albeit at their own rate and often in incremental fashion). By espousing expectation of eventual success, the practitioner's role as supportive teacher actually builds a patient's own perception of capabilities for performance (Corah 1988). If people with developmental disorders have less ability to cope with dental treatment, our goal is to help them increase their socially appropriate coping strategies (Allen et al. 1992).

Dental treatment is inherently intrusive and sometimes transiently painful (Kemp 2005). Many people become anxious and fearful at the thought of visiting the dentist, yet most develop an ability to cope with ("endure, if not enjoy") clinical dental treatment (Kemp 2005). The basic tenet of behavioral support for persons with developmental disorders is a belief/expectation that with help and guidance, they can learn to endure (cope with clinical dental treatment). Fear and anxiety are purely psychological in nature and are considered to be learned either from experience during medical or dental procedures or as a result of observed parental anxiety (Udin 1988b; Do 2004). People with developmental disorders typically have increased need for medical treatment and may have experienced multiple medical procedures prior to initial entry to the dental office. One study of children with intellectual disabilities suggested that achieving a mental age of 29 months was the delineating factor in acceptance of dental treatment (Rud & Kisling 1973). Traditional pediatric theory describes 30–36 months as the age at which a neurotypical child has developed the needed skills to respond positively to dental treatment (Festa et al. 1993). This relative agreement demonstrates a correlation between behavioral support in children and people with developmental disorders. In other words, young children and many individuals with developmental delays have the potential to or are in the process of developing coping skills to deal with stressful situations. The skillful dental practitioner can facilitate the development of those skills in both populations.

# A PEDIATRIC FOCUS

The primary principles of behavioral support for dentistry have their origins in the pediatric approach, where the goals are to create a means to communicate, limit patient anxiety, and build a trusting attitude toward dentistry while providing quality dental treatment (AAPD 2006b). A majority of dental and psychological studies examining dental fear and anxiety are focused on children, as this is the time in human development when we hopefully develop skills that allow tolerance of clinical care. Because of this behavioral focus, it is no wonder that pediatric dentists have been asked (or even expected) to provide the majority of care for children and adults with developmental disorders. However, many in the pediatric dental community now believe the role of caring for adults with developmental disorders should be taken on by general dentistry (Dougherty et al. 2001). With the advent of deinstitutionalization and extended life expectancies, this belief is undoubtedly true.

Whereas the American Dental Association (ADA), in its guidelines on control of anxiety, recognizes three behavioral methods (anxiety management, relaxation technique, and systematic desensitization), it concentrates, almost exclusively, on the use and training requirements for advanced pharmacological behavior management and accepted administration of sedation/anesthesia (ADA 2007). In contrast, the pediatric dental approach provides practitioners with the foundation for teaching patients appropriate coping mechanisms during dental treatment. Pediatric techniques have two main objectives: to establish or maintain communication between dentist and patient (necessary for learning) and to extinguish inappropriate behaviors (hopefully to be replaced by growth in cooperative skills) (AAPD 2006b). The AAPD "Guideline on Behavior Guidance for the Pediatric Patient" describes six concepts as basic approaches to behavioral support: *voice control, nonverbal communication, tell-show-do, positive reinforcement, distraction,* and *parental presence/absence.* Additional terms and interrelated strategies described in the literature include the following: *modeling, shaping, flexibility, foreshadowing, visualization, relaxation, consistency, desensitization, contingent escape, hypnosis, repetitive tasking,* and *escape extinction* (Feigal 2001; Do 2004; Tesini & Fetter 2004; Kemp 2005). Each of these concepts has potential applicability to children *and* people with developmental disorders.

# BEHAVIORAL GUIDANCE: A CLINICAL ART FORM BUILT ON SCIENTIFIC PRINCIPLES

The AAPD states that behavioral support "is a clinical art form and skill built on a foundation of science" (AAPD 2006b). Without a firm base and understanding of basic human psychology and behavior, administration of behavioral support technique is likely to be ineffective. Furthermore, failure to thoroughly understand the principles of behavioral support can actually lead to iatrogenic negative behavioral response or precipitate increased patient anxiety and noncompliance (Weinstein et al. 1982, Feigal 2001).

# ESSENTIAL TECHNIQUES OF BEHAVIORAL SUPPORT

Dental psychological science describes the following concepts, approaches, and principles as the tools the dental practitioner must be familiar with in order to effectively behaviorally support patients. Unfortunately, few have been even marginally studied in relationship to persons with developmental disorders and dentistry. Virtually none are effective independent of the others. Many overlap in their similarities or seem to be interrelated in their objectives. All require multidimensional application during the course of support of human behavior. And unlike the predictable restoration of a static, "ideal carious lesion," behavioral support of patient behavior usually involves a constantly changing treatment focus that seldom presents in an ideal fashion! A description and discussion of each technique or principle is offered, but with experience, each practitioner will develop his or her own degree of skill and finesse in use of these approaches.

- *Voice control* describes alterations of vocal volume, pace, and intonation to gain a patient's attention and influence behavioral direction (AAPD 2006b). Although communication at a level appropriate to the individual is key to behavioral support, this technique is not as much about the *message* (words) as the *means* of delivery. People with developmental disorders may have unpredictable ability to comprehend language, but most are quite adept at sensing the mood of others during interactions. Variation in delivery of spoken communication can relay temperament and acceptance (approving parent), gain patient attention and focus (lowered volume, "secret whisper"), redirect negative/avoidance behavior ("voice of God"), relax and soothe ("jazz station DJ"), direct and provide warning ("alert crossing guard"), and/or coach and create trust ("comforting friend").

  Additional communication insight: patients with developmental disorders typically have receptive communication skills that exceed their expressive skills. This means they may understand every word or the intent of everything the dental team says, though it may not be immediately evident. In the absence of functional communication skills, the practitioner must respect that behavior is patient communication in its own fashion.
- The skilled dental team recognizes when to rely on a *single voice* to communicate with the patient, as the patient may either have limited ability to process duplicative input or perceives the input as chaos from which they can escalate further disruption. Finally, it may be prudent to explain the intent of communication strategies to parents to avoid later misinterpretation.
- *Nonverbal communication* recognizes that patients may be equally or even more sensitive to touch, body language, and facial expression than to spoken language (Kemp 2005). For many people with developmental disorders, nonverbal communication may be the primary means of sensing and reading the intentions of others and interpreting situations during daily socialization. Some may benefit from gestures or visual aids. For others, removing your mask may be beneficial in order to communicate by smile and facial expression. Establishing eye contact asks the patient to focus his or her own visual attention in a personal manner. The skilled practitioner measures how he or she initiates touch (crosses into personal space) or adds physical prompts to verbal instruction (a gentle finger tap to the lower lip, to assist mouth opening). The calm, reassuring, confident actions of staff in the dental operatory will help facilitate successful behavioral support. Your words can't say one thing and your actions another: the patient will "read you like a book." Most patients will positively sense that a dental team is genuine and relaxed in their interactions. Additionally, it is important to recognize that people with developmental disorders may also use

nonverbal techniques themselves to try to control or influence their environment. The adept dental team develops its own skills of observation and learns to react to specific nonverbal cues.

- *Tell-show-do (TSD)* is the traditional approach of adding sensory demonstration cues (visual, auditory, touch, proprioception, sometimes taste/smell) to a simple verbal description of a procedure prior to performance of the procedure (Reese & Alexander 2002; AAPD 2006b). A simple example would involve showing a person the handpiece prior to letting him or her hear the whir of the rotor. Placing the prophy cup against a fingernail would then let the patient feel the vibration and tickle before starting to polish teeth. An additional step for a person with developmental disorders might include letting him or her smell the prophy paste before introducing the taste into the mouth. Even experienced patients with developmental disorders, especially those with sensory impairments, seem to benefit from continuous verbal, physical, and visual cues, as they may become distracted or startle easily with a change in stimuli. Consider the cooperative visually impaired patient who has no idea that the water spray is coming unless you let him or her know!

    "Foreshadowing" and "visualization" are similar concepts that use positive images, guided relaxation, and measured talk or play to explain to patients what to expect during new procedures or remind them that they have successfully participated in a task in the past ("remember how well you did last time") (Feigal 2001). Oftentimes, TSD provides the ancillary benefit of *educating parents* as they observe the dentist directing their child through difficult clinical treatment with positive results. If parents understand the how and why of specific behavioral approaches, they tend to become more positive and accepting of the dentist's intent and direction of support (Lawrence et al. 1991).

- *Positive reinforcement* is the process of rewarding acceptable or desired behavior with verbal praise, expression, touch, or tokens. Behaviors that are positively reinforced will increase (Kemp 2005). Positive reinforcement may be administered moment by moment throughout a procedure in an effort to direct/shape compliance during the procedure, or at the completion of major milestones during and posttreatment. For many people with developmental disorders, there is no such thing as too much positive reinforcement. In a life hindered by disability, success may be a seldom-enjoyed occurrence. Patients who have institutional or congregate living experiences (group homes, nursing homes) may find positive reinforcement in something as simple as personal recognition as an individual. Most humans crave personalized attention: voice modulation, facial expression, verbal praise, a high five, or even a smile can make a person with developmental disorders feel very exceptional. In the same way that the Special Olympian wears his or her award medal for months after an event, a small age-appropriate token, reward, or sticker can signify courage and achievement at the dental office. Consequently, this recognition of achievement serves to create self-esteem and add coping skills that will hopefully transfer to the next appointment.

- *Contingent escape* offers momentary cessation in treatment (or other positive reinforcers), conditional upon periods of acceptable target behavior (Feigal 2001; Tesini & Fetter 2004). Escape, in this technique, is used as positive reinforcement and is usually nothing more than a rest period from the stimuli (procedure). The rest period is earned (contingent) upon completion of a desired behavior (acceptable tolerance or participation in the procedure for a specific period of time) (Do 2004). The technique challenges the practitioner to monitor the patient's behavior and make judgments as to whether and when to reward escape (O'Callaghan et al. 2006).

- *Noncontingent escape* provides breaks from demands in relation to a prescribed period of time and is not dependent (contingent) upon patient compliance. This technique has been described as beneficial for children with disruptive behaviors (crying, movement, tantrums) (O'Callaghan et al. 2006). In a sense the break is not "earned," but the patient's tolerance of treatment is still rewarded regardless of behavior. A common technique used in dentistry involves counting aloud (distraction) as a promise that "we're going to rest in a second," at the same time incremental progress is being made in provision of care (Tesini & Fetter 2004).

The keys to contingent and noncontingent escape are *timing* and *honesty*. The practitioner must judge how much care (stimulus) can be completed before offering the rest period (escape). The skillful practitioner is sensitive to each individual's abilities and sets the "timer" accordingly. The second part involves the allowance of appropriate "rest/recharge time" (where the patient regroups): enough to compose him- or herself but not too long for loss of focus on task. As in all aspects of behavioral support, the practitioner must honor his or her word: *honesty builds patient trust*.

When compared, contingent reinforcement is considered superior to the noncontingent approach because there is "a vast body of evidence indicating that acquisition of new behavior is facilitated by differential consequences *contingent upon performance or nonperformance*" of desired behavior (Ingersoll et al. 1984). But the positive reinforcement offered during the rest phase in both techniques helps patients learn coping behaviors in their realization that "you know, it really wasn't that bad; in fact I guess I'm doing well because the dentist seems very happy with me!" Ultimately, this results in less disruptive behaviors, less need for advanced techniques (stabilization), and progression toward more typical and improved care.

- *Distraction* is a method of diverting a patient's mental focus to positive thoughts, favorable environmental stimuli, or other stimulating sensory images in an effort to override unpleasant procedures or as *redirection* from negative behavior (AAPD 2006b). *Passive distraction* such as pleasant sounds and smells, TV/video, or visual artwork/color designs may provide a calming atmosphere. Some individuals with developmental disorders benefit from *physical sensory distraction* such as use of a leaded x-ray apron, weighted blankets, or stabilization/hugging wraps.

Because many people with developmental disorders have shortened attention spans, they are remarkably amenable to more active distraction techniques (but the practitioner must be alert to redirect/distract behavior in a coordinated rhythm, as patient concentration wanes). As previously described, counting aloud may require the patient to focus on a mental task that "keeps his or her mind busy" while otherwise negative activity is occurring. *Imagery distraction* by storytelling, reminder of an approaching rest period, or prompted breathing exercises may otherwise divert attention. A patient's favorite music CD can concentrate the mind on something familiar and comforting and can replace a tantrum with relaxation. The skilled dental team makes an effort to discover topics of interest or stimuli that are important to the individual, and then uses their mention to redirect escalating behavior back toward cooperative participation. Remarkably, something as simple as addressing the patient by name can redirect a patient to focus. Humor can also be effective for certain patients. When sensory overload is an issue for the patient with developmental disorders, a nonstimulating environment may be the ideal setting. Music, excessive conversation, and other distractions should be eliminated to support behavior (while the calm "single voice" directs behavior through treatment progression).

- *Parental presence/absence* is intended to utilize the parent to increase patient psychological comfort and reduce patient anxiety. This debated concept may increase communication during treatment *or sometimes* proves distractive of the dentist's attempt to seize the behavioral focus of the patient (Feigal 2001). Parental demeanor clearly affects child behavior: for example, Schecter et al. (2007) have shown that excessive parental reassurance, criticism, or apology seems to increase distress related to injections, whereas humor and distraction tend to decrease distress. Contrast the impact of family dynamics as described in the common perspective that treatment success will hinge on three elements: the practitioner's skills, the abilities of the patient, and *the desires of the parents.*

Parents of children (regardless of age) with developmental disorders may present to the dental office with a number of possible emotions or concerns that will affect how you interact with and treat their child. A child (even an adult child) with special needs often implies that there is a family with special needs (Harper 1984). Emotions common to parents are varied, but consequential: grief, shock or numbness, denial, depression, frustration, anger, guilt, and acceptance are all explicable attitudes reflective of the emotional challenges and uncertainties related to disability (Willard & Nowak 1981). The practitioner may initially need to earn a family's trust by demonstration of a caring and skillful approach (Friedlander 2005). Parental presence will allow the practitioner's messages to be delivered to parents and child simultaneously, and parents will feel part of the process of decision making (Feigal 2001). When difficult behavioral support techniques must be utilized, there should never be an attempt to hide that reality from the parents. It is better that they understand and consent to the process, or refuse a treatment approach outright, than to accuse the dentist of mistreatment. It should be made clear to parents that the dentist must maintain primary communication with the child, with parents remaining silent, as much as possible, or limiting discussion to nonprocedural topics and resisting expression of fear-provoking messages (Feigal 2001). Although most dental staff might prefer parents remain in the waiting room, current parental attitudes reflect their overwhelming interest in being present during stressful procedures (Glassman et al. 1994). When parents' expectations are unreasonable, or if they are unwilling or unable to extend effective support when asked, the practitioner must decide if care should be sought elsewhere.

- *Modeling* involves having patients observe the positive behavior of others (either a filmed or in vivo model) undergoing similar procedures proposed for the patient (Do 2004). Modeling can be thought of as observational learning and may be offered as treatment preparation (waiting area video, pretreatment therapy) or as active observation of others coping in an open bay operatory (Peltier 2009). "Participant modeling" involves active imitation or *practice* by the patient of the skills exhibited by the model (White & Davis 1974). The ultimate hope is that patients will observe coping strategies that they can add to their repertoire in managing dental anxiety.

  Although there is evidence that modeling can be effective in children and many patients with developmental disorders, it may be less effective in persons with severe disabilities who may be unaffected by the behavior of those around them (Kemp 2005). Some individuals with developmental disorders seem to be unable to sense or empathize with the moods or affects of others, and thus they are unable to see themselves relating to those viewed in a modeling scenario, whereas others, in institutional or congregate living situations, are quite adept at modeling (assimilating behaviors) as they learn to imitate the behavior of cohorts in order to gain attention or reinforcement. Finally, one study provides evidence that desensitization is more effective than "video modeling" for persons with intellectual disability (Conyers et al. 2004).

- *Shaping* is a concept inherent to most basic behavioral support techniques. It describes the proper use of positive reinforcement for *approximation* of a task or behavior (and lack of reinforcement to undesirable behavior) in the effort to guide or shape increased coping by the patient (Glassman & Miller 2003). Shaping may be as simple as encouragement, compliments, or expressed gratitude for the patient who is getting closer to desired behavior. But through variations in reinforcement, shaping also helps the patient define the boundaries and expectations of the clinical setting. Many individuals with developmental disorders actually thrive in a structured environment where "the rules" are understood, predictable, and consistently reinforced. Defined and consistent boundaries enable and somewhat simplify patient learning, and shaping provides lessons for experiential learning of "the rules."

- *Flexibility* describes the recognition of patients as unique individuals with varied abilities and temperaments. Practitioners must adapt their communicative techniques, possibly moderate office tempo or routine, and assess or even alter office environment to successfully support patient behavior (Feigal 2001). Dental care of people with developmental disorders typically is more time-consuming and can require additional staff (Nowak 1976; Stiefel 2002). Flexibility asks the practitioner to relinquish some of his or her customary practice "ritual," in much the same fashion as we ask the patient with developmental disorders to give up some of the comfort of his or her "traditional structured habits!"

- *Consistency* can be simply, but energetically, described in the fact that *patients learn what they're taught!* If a message or an expectation is inconsistently delivered, the patient is confused in his or her attempt to develop skills and may be more likely to learn undesirable behavior as a result of this conflict. For example, if one considers that the vast majority of caregivers employed in group homes turn over in the course of a year, and that most lack adequate training in behavioral support, it is no wonder that people with developmental disorders have difficulty adapting to stressful situations (or even daily toothbrushing) (Glassman et al. 1994). Patients have hundreds of individuals revolving through their lives, often resulting in unbalanced and contradictory guidance in learning and growth. But when a message or situation is repeatedly presented in simple increments and in a regularly consistent fashion, people with developmental disorders can adapt, learn, and begin to predictably function in an environment with which they've become familiar. The necessity for familiarity may translate to the same operatory, the same assistant, or even the same stuffed animal being present during treatment. The realization that patients can adapt to consistent approach is the cornerstone of "basic behavior support 101."

- *Desensitization* is a general and somewhat variably defined term in dental and behavioral literature. As a pure concept, Kemp defines desensitization as "the gradual exposure of the patient to the feared object or situation with the concurrent training of and reinforcement of relaxation as a response incompatible with anxiety or fear" (Kemp 2005). Yet almost all principles of behavioral support technique involve aspects of desensitization such that common goals for desensitization are increased compliance or reduced amount of behavioral support, restraint, or sedation needed by patients as they receive clinical dental care (Conyers et al. 2004). Although desensitization to the dental office and procedures has been shown to be effective for persons with developmental disorders, the desired end points of desensitization studies are not universally described and are highly inconsistent between studies (simulated dental exams vs. meaningful treatment) (Altabet 2002; Tesini & Fetter 2004; Conyers et al. 2004). Unfortunately, therapeutic clinical dental care often involves aversive or intrusive stimuli. These stimuli vary highly in intensity and complexity (momentary but sharp, prolonged but mild) during the course of most procedures. Clinical dental treatment always involves "violation of personal space." So conceptually, desensitization (repeated exposure/tolerance) to touch or environment is behaviorally legitimate, whereas repeated needle sticks would not be accepted or beneficial. When an aversive stimulus is unavoidably necessary as part of a procedure, upon completion it is important to provide immediate and empathetic positive attention to the patient in a fashion that compliments their tolerance of care, while also attempting to negate the perception that the aversion is punishment.

As an isolated methodology, desensitization can also be expensive in terms of time, number of staff, availability of facility, and amount of repeated efforts (Tesini & Fetter 2004; Conyers et al. 2004; Kemp 2005). Desensitization programs are also difficult to apply to broad populations due to variables unique to each individual in the population, and they may delay needed care.

Thus a distinctive yet congruent technique, "on-going desensitization programming," describes an approach where in vivo *basic behavioral support* (flooding, shaping, distraction, etc.) is mutually employed in conjunction with *advanced techniques* (sedation, stabilization) during the course of actual treatment (Connick 2000). Rather than delaying needed treatment, this approach provides a person-centered approach that guides patient compliance (experiential learning, supported growth in coping skills) with a goal to fade advanced interventions, if possible, in the future. Considering the inherent constrictions in the typical dental practice, most dentists resort to this combined in vivo desensitization approach (Connick 2000).

A final thought, but as the starting point on understanding desensitization: the *foundation of oral desensitization* (and oral health) begins with parents and caregivers accepting the responsibility of providing, assisting, or teaching tolerance of daily tooth brushing! Desensitization to oral touch is best learned as a daily stimulus, not as a semiannual event.

- *Repetitive tasking*, as described by Tesini, is a component in a desensitization model based on task analysis, where a specific task (desired behavior) is broken down into incremental components. The technique involves recurring, prompted rehearsal or shaping of compliance with those components that ultimately progress to cooperation during dental treatment (Tesini & Fetter 2004). Physical guidance, social praise, and clear expectations are utilized by members of the dental team to support patient behavior through incremental mastery of the task (Kemp 2005). Although Tesini's model was created for children with autism, it is a classic example that, as humans, "we learn what we rehearse," and repetitive tasking is an applicable technique for use with most patients with developmental disorders. Practice of task increments may occur at home with caregiver support or may be delegated to dental support staff or other therapy models during desensitization appointments.

- *Hypnosis* is a method of guided self-imagery that focuses on relaxation and analgesia (Feigal 2001). It should not be purely perceived as a staged trance state but can be thought of as "a way of communicating that bypasses critical-analytical thinking" (Peltier 2009). The technique has been predominantly described and studied for use in children and adults to mediate gagging, or to overcome dental phobia, and presumes some level of patient cognizance and communicative abilities. There does not appear to be any broadly applied studies of the use of hypnosis for people with developmental disorders (Mulligan & Linderman 1979). However, many practitioners profess skill in this once traditional technique and, there are undoubtedly select patients, with mild to moderate cognitive abilities, who could benefit from the approach where structured words and sentences have a powerful impact on our patients (Peltier 2009). Most practitioners intuitively administer some degree of verbal relaxation therapy (calm, quiet tone; reassurance; and directed suggestion/distraction) and guided imagery for their anxious patients, which is often more effective when combined with use of nitrous oxide or light sedation.

- *Escape extinction* presents the counter-intuitive psychological principle that in order to overcome fear, an individual must face that fear. When a patient's disruptive behavior results in termination of (escape from) treatment, resistive behavior is reinforced and results in delay of needed care, while setting the stage for increased disruption in the future (Davis & Rombom 1979). Escape extinction, in one extreme, utilizes medical stabilization and physical guidance to provide needed treatment in response to a history of escaping treatment by physical resistance (Kemp 2005). But it may also be as simple as saying the word "no" when appropriate, or it may involve repeated verbal or physical prompting, in a way that terminates, redirects, or prohibits (fails to reinforce) escape behavior. During the course of treatment, the patient must never perceive that his or her behavior is the precipitating factor in the termination of treatment. Even when a practitioner decides that it may not be possible to complete all of the treatment planned for a specific appointment because of behavior, termination should be presented only as the operator's choice and with positive emphasis provided to the patient for his or her participation up to that point (e.g., "We have more to do next time, but you did very well today").

Flooding or *systemic desensitization* is a psychological principle that is complementary with escape extinction. It involves exposure to the fear-evoking situation (with surrounding behavioral support) until the fear subsides. In facing the fear, the patient learns that there is no reason to avoid the situation, and coping abilities are reinforced. The ethical practitioner must examine the nature of any stimulus or situation relative to an individual patient's history and characteristics: "Is this a stimulus that we are expected to learn to accept as part of our human existence?"

When basic support techniques are unsuccessful, the next generally accepted step in the hierarchy of behavioral management/support technique is a blended addition of medical immobilization/protective stabilization (MIPS) and/or pharmacologic restraint. Although protective stabilization is not a primary focus of this chapter, some discussion of this advanced methodology is included because escape extinction may rely upon a multidimensional use of behavioral support concepts and techniques in an effort to increase cooperation over time and reduce the need or degree of advanced support in the future (in vivo desensitization programming). Because MIPS is considered an advanced technique, it implies that practitioners have additional knowledge, experience, and hands-on training in its safe and effective implementation. The use of partial or complete stabilization requires that the reasons for its use are explained to the patient. Consent for use of MIPS from the guardian or patient is a legal requirement.

Finally, it is critically important that practitioners, parents, advocates and caregivers understand that the concepts of behavioral support are not terminated with the employment of more restrictive alternatives. Short of deep sedation/general anesthesia (loss of consciousness, loss of learning), the goal of behavioral support is always learned coping and progressive patient relaxation. Thus behavioral support approaches are used throughout the course of medical immobilization by a properly trained practitioner and staff. If this principle is ignored, stabilization appears more like "tie 'em up and do the work" restraint than a recognized effort at in vivo desensitization (i.e., the patient receives needed dental care assisted by protracted behavioral support, including medical stabilization) (Connick 2000). Again, there should always be an expectation of increased development of skills and consideration of possible reduction in degree of support use in the future.

# UNDERSTANDING "LIFE DYNAMICS" EFFECT ON BEHAVIOR

Although many of the behavioral support techniques available to dentistry are common to both pediatric and special needs care, there are additional and important issues that are specific to the field of care for persons with developmental disorders. As a group, people with developmental disorders represent a significantly more diverse or heterogeneous segment of the population than that treated in the pediatric dental office. Patients with developmental disorders present as both children and adults with a wide array of disabling conditions and varied degrees of severity of impairment (Stiefel 2002). Most of these issues further complicate care provision and present significant challenges for the dental team.

The life expectancy of children with disabilities is increasing (Janicki et al. 1999). Adulthood may produce growth in coping skill and cooperative behaviors. However, aging may also simply be a chronological event, which has little benefit or even detrimental effect on the overall quality of life for the person with developmental disorders. As a student with developmental disorders graduates from special education programs, he or she may suffer a cut in therapeutic behavioral support services. At the same time, in most states, he or she will "age out" of Medicaid dental benefit coverage (Waldman & Perlman 1997). This may result in less routine dental visits, which may lead to decreased carryover of learned skills and increased resistance, not to mention advancement of oral disease.

The practical reality is that the person with developmental disorders may spend much of his or her life in an atmosphere of unpredictable chaos. Over a lifetime individual living situations are often unsettled, inconsistent, and challenging (familial dysfunction/stress, multiple group homes, possible institutionalizations, challenged peers/roommates). Support staff and caregivers turn over at an astronomical rate, such that trusted relationships are difficult to establish, ever changing, and repeatedly and sadly lost. Most will rely on others to meet some or all of their daily needs, as well as to report/describe medical, behavioral, and social conditions (e.g., "The van driver has no idea how I feel, what has occurred in my life, or what I'm trying to communicate!"). And many will be treated by multiple physicians who, although well meaning, may prescribe multiple medications that may not be compatible and/or beneficial to function and quality of life.

Other factors related to behavioral support demands for patients with developmental disorders as they age into adulthood include the following:

- Behavioral resistance exhibited by an adult may have more dramatic consequences than similar behavior in a 3-year-old!
- Parents of children with developmental disorders may not seek access to dental treatment until later in their child's life, due to pressing medical and developmental concerns that pervade the childhood years (Pilcher 1997). Parents may also be apprehensive about finding a dentist who will treat their child or are nervous as to how their child will behave in the dental chair. After many unsuccessful attempts to find a dentist to treat their child, they simply give up. Because of this delay, there is greater likelihood that a patient has built up anxiety as a result of multiple medical encounters or has developed fear of dentistry, transferred from familial attitudes or input from siblings and peers (Wright 1975). As a result, dental disease may have progressed and treatment needs may be excessive (Glassman & Miller 2003).

- As a result of the above factors, people with developmental disorders often initially present to the dental office with emergent treatment needs. There is no more difficult a situation for the dental team and patient than to initiate a relationship under the cloud of acute pain, infection, and possibly complex surgical demands. The practitioner is challenged to utilize all of his or her behavioral support skills, but it is likely that all involved players will remember the encounter as an aversive and difficult event. (Contrast this example with the ideal behavioral treatment planning process, where initial treatment focuses on completion of the least demanding procedure in order to desensitize and shape cooperative success.)
- Patients with developmental disorders who have experienced institutional and other congregate living situations may present with behaviors that are modeled from observing the disruptive actions of their peers. These behaviors may be learned out of a common environmental need (attention seeking, escape, self-stimulation) or may simply be adaptive imitation of the "surrounding culture."
- People with developmental disorders are exceedingly vulnerable to exploitation and neglect and are estimated to suffer abuse at the hands of others at a rate 10 times greater than that of the general population (Burtner & Dicks 1994; Sobsey 1994). This fact complicates aspects of trying to interpret patient behavior when dentistry, by its nature, demands violation of personal space. What appears to be a noncompliant tantrum may actually be posttraumatic stress disorder reflective of a prior abusive experience.
- Mental illness (psychiatric disorders) occurs more commonly in persons with intellectual disability than in the general population (Szymanski & King 1999). Clinical presentation, diagnosis, and treatment of the mental disorder is often complicated by poor language and cognitive skill inherent in a dual diagnosis.
- With extended life expectancy, persons with developmental disorders face an increased risk/incidence of acquired geriatric disabilities (functional and sensory) (Ettinger & Kambhu 1992; Arias 2004). When sensory loss affects changes in intelligence, memory, and learning ability, the loss of cognitive function creates new dilemmas in the behavioral support of the geriatric patient with developmental disorders. Although Alzheimer's disease, the most common form of dementia, occurs in approximately 11% of Americans over age 65, it is estimated that 25% or more of individuals with Down syndrome over age 35 show clinical signs and symptoms of Alzheimer's-type dementia (Little 2005). The incidence of Alzheimer's disease in the Down syndrome population is estimated to be 3–5 times greater than in the general population, and oftentimes symptoms begin much earlier. Dementia initially impairs cognitive function and later results in impaired behaviors (California Statewide Taskforce on Oral Health 2005). The geriatric patient with developmental disorders creates a new dilemma for dentistry in that

the coping skills that may have been honed through relationship and support are now in flux and are erratically on the decline (Carr-Hosie 1993). Fortunately, Chalmers, in her comprehensive review of geriatric behavior, reports that behavioral supports for patients with dementia utilize the same principles already described but with a slightly different focus (2000). *Flexibility* is repeated as the characteristic critical to successful care of people with dementia (Hallberg et al. 1995; Kayser-Jones et al. 1996). Techniques that work for some patients may not work for others, and what works one day for one person may not be effective the next day for the same person (Niessen et al. 1985; Kovach 1997). Dr. Janet Yellowitz, past president of the American Society of Geriatric Dentistry, aptly states that "patients with dementia not only have good days and bad days, they have good minutes and bad minutes," such that, in as little as 5 minutes, a patient may completely change his or her mood, lucidity, and ability to participate in care (*coping*) (Yellowitz, personal communication, 2006). *The topic of the "aging patient" with a developmental disorder will be discussed in more detail at the end of this chapter.*

- Because of their extensive life experience, patients with developmental disorders may develop an extensive and effective repertoire of avoidance behaviors that includes the following: behavioral gag, volitional emesis, willful voiding (or repeated false claim for bathroom—"pee pee, pee pee"), nontearful vocalization, and hysteria. (Commonsense strategies include making sure patients with gag risks are seen with an empty stomach and that patients are encouraged to visit the toilet prior to treatment.) These actions reflect adapted use of basic human functions or behavior, sometimes in sophisticated fashion, as a means to manipulate one's environment. Many patients learn well (classic conditioning) that these behaviors allow them to "get their way" or otherwise eliminate stimuli. However, it is also important to recognize that avoidance behaviors (such as vocalization, hysteria) may actually be *avoidance coping* in that they serve as a means of beneficial detachment or mental diversion of attention from present reality/stressful stimuli (Chambers 1970; Bernard et al. 2004; Peltier 2009). Remarkably, the committed dental team can work to extinguish detrimental avoidance behaviors by utilizing the basic techniques described in the literature. It takes time and perseverance and may require use of escape extinction as a strategy to establish communication, but the dental team's focus should remain unchanged: reinforce positive behaviors while ignoring or redirecting "melodramatics" (do not reward/reinforce negative behaviors). This description is not meant to sound judgmental in any way. Each of us has learned to manipulate our environment within the limits that family and society have set for us. Sometime today it is likely that each reader will theatrically "act" in some fashion in order to influence his or her environment!

- Nature versus nurture—diagnostic overshadowing occurs when a patient's problematic behaviors are attributed *solely* to their neurodevelopmental disorder (Sundheim & Ryan 1999). Dentists unfamiliar with people with developmental disorders may assume that all patient behavior is the direct result of their disability, when actually only a portion is attributable to the primary impairment. The majority of a patient's behaviors *may* be representative of his or her overall life circumstance and experience, such as parent-related stress and familial dysfunction, extent and quality of nurturing, directive consistency, and/or setting of expectations during the developmental period (Hauser-Cram et al. 2001; AAPD 2006b). Overindulgence, failure to establish boundaries, emotional abandonment, or failure to bond may "socially disable" the individual to a greater degree than the primary disability itself. Similarly, abuse or an imposed institutional culture may be evident as "psychological scarring" in the behavioral profile of the patient with developmental disorders, regardless of the form or nature of his or her primary disability.

This discussion accentuates the challenging and complex nature of the task required of the dental team to behaviorally diagnose and support a patient through the course of clinical care.

## THE "ART PART" OF BEHAVIORAL SUPPORT

*Creative energy.*
*Timing is everything!*
*Synchronization and interactive effects.*

There seems to be a consensus regarding distinctive characteristics most common to dentists who find care of people with developmental disorders to be rewarding. They are typically described as having a high degree of empathy, patience, and compassion and a friendly and caring demeanor (Willard & Nowak 1981; Stiefel 2002; Glassman et al. 2004; Kemp 2005; AAPD 2006b; Casamassimo 2006). The practitioner who is willing to be flexible about the usually stringent routines of the typical dental practice will find ways to adapt care to the needs of the patient. Another way of approaching this care is to consider "turning your typical practice mental tension level down a couple of notches" and to "be patient with your patient, patient with your staff, and patient with yourself." Something as simple as giving a patient time to process and respond to a request can produce remarkable results. Consider the contrast of a patient who will try to perform, if given time, with the patient whose behavior escalates out of frustration simply because he or she has not been given the time or a chance to comply. From a similar perspective, the practitioner who can be forgiving of patient, staff, and self will ultimately find more success and satisfaction in providing care to people with developmental disorders. Realize that everyone is probably doing the best he or she can, and profess a confidence that "it will get better" with time, as learning progresses and as relationships and familiarity grow. It may be beneficial to hold postop debriefings where dental staff may de-stress, discuss their impression of how treatment progressed (what went well, what could have gone better), and decide on strategies to improve support at subsequent appointments. A similar debriefing and reassurance may be beneficial to the patient and family or caregivers.

How does the practitioner put it all together? Few, if any, of these principles alone are sufficient to reduce uncooperative behaviors. Almost all approaches share elements from other concepts. The dentist must blend application of multiple techniques in a paced, synchronized fashion, in order to specifically support the moment-by-moment behavior of the patient (timing: attention, distraction, escape/rewards, and recharge). The skilled practitioner uses these principles much like a painter uses a color palette; all techniques are on hand to be selectively dabbed or blended into the picture to achieve precise behavioral effect. The dental staff accepts responsibility for setting up the easel and making sure that the lighting is just right (prepares the environment and reviews specific needs of the patient). The end result may not always be a masterpiece, but even a picture worth hanging on the fridge represents success!

## SCULPTING SUCCESSFUL SUPPORT STRATEGIES

*Teamwork ("four c's"): committed, calm, confident, consistent.*
*Familiar setting and staff.*
*Adequate staffing and time.*

Basic behavioral support begins at the time of the initial patient encounter, when the basic foundation of a *relationship* is poured, and when desensitization to dental treatment begins. When compared to a medical exam room (minimal stimuli, benign atmosphere), the typical dental operatory may appear threatening and perplexing (Glassman et al. 2004). Thus, experts in dental and psychology literature suggest eliminating environmental stressors by using the practitioner's private office or an interview room to perform the initial patient medical and behavior assessment (Glassman et al. 2004; Kemp 2005). An empty waiting room, set aside for a new patient intake, can prove to be a spacious, nonthreatening setting where socialization can occur. In this setting, the dental team can join to observe fundamental patient behavioral characteristics during the course of the often extensive health history review. This is also a time when the practitioner and each staff member should meet and focus on the patient, addressing him or her by name and establishing eye contact (if possible). The intent is to express welcome and acceptance and to acknowledge the patient's identity as an individual of importance. To further this intent and build trust, whenever possible, efforts should be made to communicate directly with the patient (Pilcher 1997). A socially acceptable degree of touch (handshake, shoulder pat, "high five," etc.) will establish the concept that dental care will require touch and necessitates some "violation of personal space." Tactile defensiveness, if present, will become evident in the course of this encounter.

Other important characteristics that deserve evaluation during the initial interview include assessment of socialization skills, degree of possible sensory impairment, cognitive level, and attention span. The dental team should also discover the degree to which the patient's receptive and expressive communicative levels vary (Pilcher 1997). Waiting times should also be minimized as much as possible in order to reduce patient tension (Chalmers 2000).

Research has established that mental age is a greater determinant of acceptance of treatment than chronological age (Udin 1988a). Thus an honest assessment of a patient's cognitive or functional level may be vital to the provision of appropriate behavioral support and communication technique (Kemp 2005). Such assessment will guide the practitioner in sculpting individualized patient care that reflects each patient's stage of development and level of coping and learning skills. The practitioner's intent is to help the patient with developmental disorders through a stressful situation at a level that meets his or her needs but doesn't seek to negate the concept of "age appropriateness" in overall personal dignity and respect. Finally, gaining some measure of the length of an individual's attention span will help the practitioner design treatment strategies, while formulating a treatment plan.

Reflective of, or unrelated to, attention span, each person with developmental disorders has what might be called a "cooperative window" that reflects how long he or she can stay in the "cooperative ballpark." For many, there appears to be a predictable period of time where they can muster their coping skills and tolerate or allow treatment. But when that time is used up, they seem to say "I can't play anymore," and behavior tends to deteriorate. A practitioner who learns to respect this phenomenon will likely guide the patient through numerous successful treatment encounters. The dentist who insists on completing the quadrant because "that's the way I do things" will likely damage the trust of the patient and iatrogenically precipitate increased resistance at future appointments simply because the patient's cooperative efforts weren't respected.

Nowhere else in dentistry is *"teamwork"* more critical than when providing behavioral support to people with developmental disorders. Because many people with developmental disorders are keenly adept at reading nonverbal cues, they more readily sense anxiety or uncertainty in individual staff members (*show no fear*: "we've seen this before and we're here to help you!"). The patient may exploit any perceived "weak link" to try to manipulate or disrupt proposed treatment. A special care team that presents itself as *calmly confident, consistent*, and *committed* to successful treatment will actually discover it can guide a patient through treatment, where other clinicians have failed. This confident team carries an expectation that it can discover a means to support the patient in some fashion that will provide for meaningful care. Such a staff creates a "circle of behavioral support" that is consistent in its message, thus facilitating patient learning and development of enhanced coping skills.

Because persons with developmental disorders find comfort in familiar settings, try to treat a patient in the same operatory with members of the staff that they've met before. Additionally, patients will often appear more at ease and less stressed with a favored caregiver or the more supportive parent. When possible, schedule appointments that allow the most trusted and confident team member to accompany the patient: *supportive relationships strengthen our coping skills.*

In a similar fashion, it is critical that family or caregivers continue to bolster this learning postoperatively by responding in positive terms and providing reinforcing attention for a job well done. Nothing undermines positive behavioral growth more effectively than a parent/caregiver who greets a patient with a "my poor baby—what did they do to you" attitude in the waiting area after that patient has worked hard to participate during treatment. The patient becomes confused, one minute being regaled for his or her coping behavior, the next minute receiving sympathy for what must have been a "horrible event." Thus the dental team's expectation for success must also be transferred to family and caregivers, in order to reinforce continued behavioral growth. A dental team should find it rewarding to share in a celebration of accomplishment with a patient and his or her family; *such accomplishments are the seeds of self-esteem.* This perpetuates the concept that consistency, in message and method, helps people with developmental disorders learn to cope during stressful events.

# ADVANCED TECHNIQUE: SEDATION AND GENERAL ANESTHESIA

In order to provide the best appropriate care to patients with developmental disorders, a dental care system or community should be able to utilize or access all possible methodologies in the hierarchy of behavioral support techniques. Although dentistry currently seems to have placed most of its focus on the *pharmacological management of patient behavior and anxiety,* organized dentistry and many state boards have increasingly placed limitations on the use of preoperative and in-office sedation and anesthesia. Thus many practitioners are less willing to provide this service, which creates an additional barrier to access for patients who might benefit from its use. And because medical procedures typically generate more income for a hospital than dental procedures, dentists in many parts of the country are finding it increasingly difficult to schedule operating room time to treat patients with developmental disorders (California Statewide Taskforce on Oral Health 2005).

Considering this lengthy discussion of the importance of basic behavioral support, which is generally considered to have fewer side effects than pharmacologic intervention, there are admittedly classic situations where general anesthesia is the best alternative. When a dental team cannot assure the physical safety of the patient or staff, deep sedation or anesthesia is an obvious and necessary treatment alternative. Even for the patient who can be treated using basic behavioral support techniques, there may be certain procedures, such as complicated extractions, that would best be performed with a patient "asleep." There will be certain medically compromised or delicate patients who may be more safely monitored and less stressed with treatment in the operating room. Some patients who may ultimately benefit from behavioral support may initially present with emergent needs that cannot wait for desensitization. And sometimes practical issues such as extreme disease, cost of parental time away from work, difficulties with extraordinary scheduling demands, or great distance and/or transportation burdens may force the dentist to recommend comprehensive care utilizing the assistance of the anesthesiologist. So a very justifiable use for general anesthesia would be for the full mouth rehabilitation of a rampantly diseased mouth in one session, *even when long-term care and maintenance of a patient may be achievable using simple behavioral support techniques.* And in a final contrast, an advantage of anesthesia may be a relative amnesia of much of the event, although any potential for developing relationships and patient learning and growth of coping skills is negated using this approach.

## SUMMARY

Dentistry's focus on behavioral support is profoundly based on pediatric concept, approach, and technique. The pediatric dentist is trained and skilled in the behavioral guidance of children during clinical dental treatment. Similarly, the practitioner who cares for people with developmental disorders must possess a spectrum of skills founded in the concept of communicative learning, but those skills must be further adapted, perfected, and applied to a much more heterogeneous segment of humanity than children alone. The patient with developmental disorders typically presents to the dental office with a more complex behavioral profile, a broader life experience, a multitude of prior medical encounters, and a possible history of congregate living arrangements and is more likely to have been a victim of abuse than a child patient. Patients with developmental disorders should be perceived as having potential for cognitive growth/learning and recognized as individuals with unique human personalities who share our common needs.

Skillful application of behavioral support techniques is somewhat intuitive and empirical. It is as much an art form as it is a science. Unlike many procedures in dentistry, there is no universal formula or simplistic step-by-step diagram for practitioners to follow in the application of behavioral support techniques for the broad spectrum of individuals with developmental disorders. Some practitioners are artists while others aren't; there is no easily defined standard for performance. Dental practitioners who treat people with developmental disorders typically possess a unique temperament and possibly a holistic view of dentistry's intertwined relationship with psychology and human behavior. Success in treating people with developmental disorders depends on allowing additional time, having adequate trained staff, and creating an environment that the patient can recognize as familiar. Caring for people with developmental disorders can be physically and emotionally demanding and requires patience and a vision of sculpted behavioral support for a patient who may perceive treatment to be aversive and threatening. The degree to which people with developmental disorders will be relegated to treatment utilizing deep sedation or general anesthesia may be more dependent on a practitioner's skill and commitment to developing a trusted relationship using behavioral support techniques than on the unique presenting characteristics of the patient. Using these described techniques in a skilled and thoughtful fashion may require more time and patience from the dental team, but the results can be dramatic and rewarding.

# REFERENCES

Allen KD, Loiben T, Allen SJ, Stanley RT. (1992). Dentist-implemented contingent escape for management of disruptive child behavior. *Journal of Applied Behavioral Analysis* 25(3):629–636.

Altabet SC. (2002). Decreasing dental resistance among individuals with severe and profound mental retardation. *Journal of Developmental and Physical Disabilities* 14(3):297–305.

American Academy of Pediatric Dentistry (AAPD). (2006a). Clinical Affairs Committee—Behavior Management Subcommittee; American Academy of Pediatric Dentistry Council on Clinical Affairs—Committee on Behavior Guidance (2005–2006). Guideline on behavior guidance for the pediatric patient. *Pediatric Dentistry* 27(7 Reference Manual):92–100.

———. (2006b). Council on Clinical Affairs Committee (2005–2006). Guideline on management of persons with special health care needs. *Pediatric Dentistry*, 27(7 Reference Manual):80–83.

American Dental Association (ADA). (2007). Guidelines for teaching the comprehensive control of anxiety and pain in dentistry. As adopted by the October 2007 American Dental Association's House of Delegates, Chicago, IL.

Arias E. (2004). United States life tables 2002. *National Vital Statistics Reports* 53(6):1–38.

Bernard RS, Cohen LL, McClellan CB, et al. (2004). Pediatric procedural approach-avoidance coping and distress: A multitrait-multimethod analysis. *Journal of Pediatric Psychology* 29(2):131–141.

Burtner AP, Dicks JL. (1994). Providing oral health care to individuals with severe disabilities residing in the community: Alternative delivery systems. *Special Care in Dentistry* 14:188–193.

California Statewide Taskforce on Oral Health for People with Developmental Disorders and the Statewide Taskforce on Oral Health and Aging Policy Reform Agenda. (2005). October 14.

Carr-Hosie MA. (1993). Treatment considerations for the dental profession for patients with Alzheimer's disease. *Journal of the Oklahoma Dental Association* 83(3):36–42.

Casamassimo PS. (2006). Children with special health care needs; patient, professional and systemic issues (Pediatric Oral Health Interfaces Background Paper). Accessed May 1, 2006, from http://www.cdhp.org/downloads/interfaces/interfaces%20special%20health%20care.pdf#search=%22Children%20with%20special%20health%20care%20needs%3B%20patient%2C%20professional%20and%20systemic%20issues%22.

Casamassimo PS, Seale NS, Ruehs K. (2004). General dentists' perceptions of educational and treatment issues affecting access to care for children with special health care needs. *Journal of Dental Education* 68(1):23–28.

Chalmers JM. (2000). Behavior management and communication strategies for dental professional when caring for patients with dementia. *Special Care in Dentistry* 20(4):147–154.

Chambers DW. (1970). Managing the anxieties of young dental patients. *Journal of Dentistry for Children* 37:363–374.

Clevenger WE, Wigal T, Salvati N, et al. (1993). Dental needs of persons with developmental disabilities in Orange County. *Journal of Developmental and Physical Disabilities* 5:253–264.

Connick CM. (2000). Appropriate use of restraint with on-going desensitization programming. *Interface* 16(3):4.

Conyers C, Miltenberger RG, Peterson B, et al. (2004). An evaluation of in vivo desensitization and video modeling to increase compliance with dental procedures in persons with mental retardation. *Journal of Applied Behavioral Analysis* 37(2):233–238.

Corah NL. (1988). Dental anxiety: Assessment, reduction and increasing patient satisfaction. *Dental Clinics of North America* 32(4):779–790.

Davis MJ, Rombom HM. (1979). Survey of the utilization of and rationale for hand-over-mouth (HOM) and restraint in postdoctoral education. *Pediatric Dentistry* 1:87–90.

Do C. (2004). Applying the social learning theory to children with dental anxiety. *Journal of Contemporary Dental Practice* (5)1:126–135.

Dougherty N, Romer M, Lee RS. (2001). Trends in special care training in pediatric dental residencies. *ASDC Journal of Dentistry for Children* 68(5–6): 384–387, 303.

Ettinger RL, Kambhu PP. (1992). Selected issues on care and management of the ageing patient: 1. Utilization and decision making. *Dental Update* 19(5):208–212.

Feigal RJ. (2001). Guiding and managing the child dental patient: A fresh look at old pedagogy. *Journal of Dental Education* 65(12):1369–1377.

Fenton SJ, Fenton LI, Kimmelman BB, et al. (1987). ADH ad hoc committee report: The use of restraints in the delivery of dental care for the handicapped—legal, ethical, and medical considerations. *Special Care in Dentistry* 7(6):253–256.

Festa SA, Ferguson FS, Hauk M. (1993). Behavior management techniques in pediatric dentistry. *New York State Dental Journal* 59(2):35–38.

Friedlander AH. (2005). Autism: Acknowledging the heritable aspects of illness as possible barriers to successfully marshalling family assistance. *Special Care in Dentistry* 25(4):177.

Friedlander AH, Yagiela JA, Paterno VI, et al. (2003). The pathophysiology, medical management, and dental implications of autism. *Journal of the California Dental Association* 31(9):681–691.

Glassman P, Henderson T, Helgeson M, et al. (2005). Oral health for people with developmental disorders: Consensus statement on implications and recommendations for the dental profession. *Journal of the California Dental Association* 33(8):619–623.

Glassman P, Miller C. (2003). Dental disease prevention and people with developmental disorders. *Journal of the California Dental Association* 31(3):257–269.

Glassman P, Miller C, Ingraham R, et al. (2004). The extraordinary vulnerability of people with disabilities: Guidelines for oral health professionals. *Journal of the California Dental Association* 32(5):379–386.

Glassman P, Miller C, Wozniak T, et al. (1994). A preventive dentistry training program for caretakers of persons with disabilities residing in community residential facilities. *Special Care in Dentistry* 14:137–143.

Gordon SM, Dionne RA, Snyder J. (1998). Dental fear and anxiety as a barrier to accessing oral health care among patients with special health care needs. *Special Care in Dentistry* 18(2):88–92.

Governor's Commission on Mental Retardation. (1994). Strategies for change: Supporting persons with mental retardation who have health and behavioral challenges. Boston: Commonwealth of Massachusetts. Accessed Sept. 28, 2008, from http://www.mass.gov/gcmr/pdf/Strategies_Health_Behavioral_ Challanges.pdf.

Griffen AL, Schneiderman LJ. (1992). Ethical issues in managing the noncompliant child. *Pediatric Dentistry* 14(3):178–183.

Hallberg IR, Holst G, Nordmark A, et al. (1995). Cooperation during morning care between nurses and severely demented institutionalized patients. *Clinical Nursing Research* 4:78–104.

Harper DC. (1984). Child behavior toward the parent: A factor analysis of mothers' reports of disabled children. *Journal of Autism and Developmental Disorders* 14(2):165–182.

Hauser-Cram P, Warfield ME, Shonkoff JP, et al. (2001). Children with disabilities: A longitudinal study of child development and parent well-being. *Monographs of the Society for Research in Child Development* 66(3):i–viii, 1–114, discussion 115–126.

Ingersoll BD, Nash DA, Blount RI, et al. (1984). Distraction and contingent reinforcement with pediatric dental patients. *ASDC Journal of Dentistry for Children* 51:203–207.

Janicki MP, Dalton AJ, Henderson CM, et al. (1999). Mortality and morbidity among older adults with intellectual disability: Health services considerations. *Disability and Rehabilitation* 21:284–294.

Kayser-Jones J, Bird WF, Redford M, et al. (1996). Strategies for conducting dental examinations among cognitively impaired nursing home residents. *Special Care in Dentistry* 16:46–52.

Kemp F. (2005). Alternatives: A review of non-pharmacologic approaches to increasing the cooperation of patients with developmental disorders to inherently unpleasant dental procedures. *Behavior Analyst Today* 6(2):88–108.

Kovach CR. (1997). *Late-Stage Dementia Care: A Basic Guide*. Washington, DC: Taylor & Francis.

Lawrence SM, McTigue DJ, Wilson S, et al. (1991). Parental attitudes toward behavior management techniques used in pediatric dentistry. *Pediatric Dentistry* 13:151–155.

Little JW. (2005). Dental management of patients with Alzheimer's disease. *General Dentistry* 53(4):289–296.

Lyons RA. (2004). Dentistry's dilemma: Adults with developmental disorders. *Pediatric Dentistry Today* 40:30.

Mulligan R, Lindeman R. (1979). Behavior modification utilizing hypnosis in a minimal brain dysfunction patient. *Journal of Dentistry for the Handicapped* 4(2):41–43.

Niessen LC, Jones JA, Zocchi M, et al. (1985). Dental care for the patient with Alzheimer's disease. *Journal of the American Dental Association* 110:207–209.

Nowak AJ. (1976). *Dentistry for the Handicapped Patient*. St. Louis: Mosby.

O'Callaghan PM, Allen KD, Powell S, et al. (2006). The efficacy of noncontingent escape for decreasing children's disruptive behavior during restorative dental treatment. *Journal of Applied Behavioral Analysis* 39(2):161–171.

Peltier B. (2009). Psychological treatment of fearful and phobic special needs patients. *Special Care in Dentistry* 29(1):51–57.

Peretz B, Glaicher H, Ram D. (2003). Child-management techniques: Are there differences in the way female and male pediatric dentists in Israel practice? *Brazilian Dental Journal* 14(2):82–86.

Pilcher ES. (1997). Dental care for the patient with Down syndrome. Paper presented at the 6th World Congress on Down Syndrome, October 1–6, Madrid, Spain.

Reese RG, Alexander M. (2002). Managing child behaviors in the dental setting. *Clinical Update* (Naval Postgraduate Dental School) 24(7). Accessed from http://www.bethesda.med.navy.mil/careers/postgraduate_dental_school/research/.

Romer M, Dougherty N, Amores-LaFleur E. (1999). Predoctoral education in special care dentistry: Paving the way to better access? *ASDC Journal of Dentistry for Children* 66:132–135.

Rud B, Kisling E. (1973). The influence of mental development on children's acceptance of dental treatment. *Scandinavian Journal of Dental Research* 81:343–352.

Schecter NL, Zempsky WT, Cohen LL, et al. (2007). Pain reduction during pediatric immunizations: Evidence-based review and recommendations. *Pediatrics* 119(5):1184–1198.

Sobsey D. (1994). *Violence and Abuse in the Lives of People with Disabilities: The End of Silent Acceptance?* Baltimore: Paul H. Brookes Publishing Co.

Southern Association of Institutional Dentists (SAID). (2001a). *Clinical Concerns in the Provision of Dental Care for Clients with Mental Retardation.* SAID Self Study Course: Module 2: 1–8. Accessed December 12, 2010, from http://www.saiddent.org/modules/10_module2.pdf.

———. (2001b). *Managing Maladaptive Behaviors: The Use of Dental Restraints and Positioning Devices.* SAID Self Study Course: Module 6: 1–24. Accessed December 12, 2010, from http://www.saiddent.org/modules/14_module6.pdf.

Stiefel DJ. (2002). Dental care considerations for disabled adults. *Special Care in Dentistry* 22(3):26S–39S.

Subarian SR. (2001). Developmental disabilities and understanding the needs of patients with mental retardation and Down syndrome. *Journal of the California Dental Association* 29(6):415–423.

Sundheim ST, Ryan RM. (1999). Amnestic syndrome presenting as malingering in a man with developmental disability. *Psychiatric Services* 50:966–968.

Szymanski L, King BH. (1999). Practice parameters for the assessment and treatment of children, adolescents, and adults with mental retardation and comorbid mental disorders. American Academy of Child and Adolescent Psychiatry Working Group on Quality Issues. *Journal of the American Academy of Child and Adolescent Psychiatry* 38(12):5S–31S.

Tesini D, Fetter C. (2004). *D-Termined Program of Repetitive Tasking and Familiarization in Dentistry.* Hampton, NH: Specialized Care Co. [DVD].

Thierer T, Meyerowitz C. (2005). Education of dentists in the treatment of patients with developmental disorders. *Journal of the California Dental Association* 33(9):723–729.

Udin RD. (1988a). Assessing dental manageability of handicapped children. *Journal of Pedodontics* 13(1):29–37.

———. (1988b). Predictors of dental behavior of disabled children. *Journal of Pedodontics* 12(3):250–259.

Waldman HB, Perlman SP. (1997). Children with disabilities are aging out of dental care. *ASDC Journal of Dentistry for Children* 64(6):385–390.

Weinstein P, Getz T, Ratener P, Domoto P. (1982). The effect of dentist's behavior on fear-related behaviors in children. *Journal of the American Dental Association* 104:32–38.

White WC, Davis MT. (1974). Vicarious extinction of phobic behavior in early childhood. *Journal of Abnormal Psychology* 2(1):25–32.

Willard DH, Nowak AJ. (1981). Communicating with the family of the child with a developmental disability. *Journal of the American Dental Association* 102:647–650.

Wright GZ. (1975). *Behavior Management in Dentistry for Children.* Philadelphia: Saunders.

Yellowitz JA, Dunhoff KL, Smith KA. (2004). Caring for the elderly—special care dentistry. *Pennsylvania Dental Journal* 71(1):36–40.

# Section 2: Alternative behavioral support strategies

Clive Friedman, DDS

## ALTERNATIVE BEHAVIOR STRATEGIES

In the first section of this chapter, Dr. Lyons discusses a team that is not familiar with strategies for successfully accommodating behavior and how this can impede its ability to provide care. This section will outline a few strategies for accommodating behaviors that would not normally be considered within the confines of a daily practice, which may widen this perspective.

Processes facilitated by other therapists, such as music, craniosacral, and equine therapy, as well as those that can be carried out by the dental team, including sensory integration and social stories, are offered as additive methods for use as the practitioner develops his or her own approach.

Dr. Lyons details communication strategies and highlights the importance of connecting to the patient. He explains how theories, techniques, or processes do not work if the practitioner does not connect with the patient first. Dan Siegel, in his book *The Mindful Therapist* (2010), presents a model that is useful in combining many of the thoughts described in the previous section. He discusses in detail what is required to both connect to the patient and, just as importantly, to connect to one's own internal process. When the practitioner is distracted by the challenges in his or her own life, it is very difficult to be completely present for the patient he or she should be working with. Most health care professionals trained in the medical model tend to view themselves as the expert and have a need to fix a

*Treating the Dental Patient with a Developmental Disorder*, First Edition.
Edited by Karen A. Raposa and Steven P. Perlman.
© 2012 John Wiley & Sons, Inc. Published 2012 by John Wiley & Sons, Inc.

person's problem. They perceive that people do not change because they have a lack of knowledge, insight, capability, or motivation and have a need to make this right. Miller and Rollnick (2002) describe this as a "deficit worldview." A radical shift in thinking to a worldview of "competency" would view individuals as having everything they need and being their own experts. This approach is collaborative and honors an individual's autonomy. Presence depends on a sense of safety. The brain continually monitors the external and internal environment for signs of danger in a process called "neuroception." When danger is felt it goes on high alert or the fight or flight response is activated (amygdala attack). This response involves the prefrontal, limbic, and brainstem processes and is shaped by historical experiences. If things are seen as threatening, then the open space of possibility is left for the reactive fight or freeze response. Simply forcing a child to have his or her teeth brushed could evoke such a response. One can imagine many similar experiences in the dental situation, thus it is important to be aware of this response both in the patient as well as in oneself. If one's own amygdala is alerted, it does not allow one to be present. By being fully present to individuals with disabilities, the practitioner would be aware when the amygdala is stimulated and be able to back off and reevaluate his or her approach. Siegel provides excellent tools to help each member of a team to not only identify when this is happening but also to overcome it. Being mindful of the different nuances and approaches to care with individuals with developmental disabilities is not always simple, but with awareness it can shift the process to one of ease and joy.

## SENSORY-ADAPTED ENVIRONMENTS

Individuals with developmental disabilities have a variety of sensory impediments. They may be hyper- or hyposensitive to touch, smells, hearing, taste, or sound. They will often have difficulty sensing where one's body is in a given space. In a dental office environment these senses are very much a part of an individual's experience. Being sensitive to and creating an atmosphere that will integrate or decrease the impact of these senses might help the individual cope with invasive dental procedures. (See Appendix 4.2.1 for a form to help alert the team to these issues.) The brains of individuals with special needs seem to be unable to balance the senses appropriately and filter stimuli and thus may be subjected to overwhelming amounts of sensory input on a continual basis (Iarocci & McDonald 2006). Thus, where possible, creating an environment that is conducive to helping minimize excess stimulation is advisable.

### Environmental changes

Minimizing excess stimuli can be as simple as using a separate room that is quiet and has subdued lighting, relaxing music, or even running water.

Shapiro et al. (2009) have shown how these environmental changes decrease anxiety. More elaborate and expensive technologies like Snoezelen have also been shown to reduce anxiety and calm individuals with sensory impairments. Snoezelen can be staged to provide a multisensory experience or single sensory focus, simply by adapting the lighting, atmosphere, sounds, and textures to the specific needs of the client at the time of use. It has been used with success in many hospital environments.

## Aroma therapy

Smell is the only sense that bypasses the central cortex and goes directly to the amygdala. It is not therefore uncommon for an array of emotions to be triggered by smells of dental offices or hospitals. Smells can condition patients negatively toward dental care. Many individuals with disabilities will react not only when seeing a building but also when entering it, and it may be impossible to get the person into the office. Lehrner et al. (2005), in their study on reducing anxiety in the dental office, showed how the use of odors such as lavender or orange reduces anxiety and improves mood. Finding alternative spaces or altering the ambient smell may be all that is needed to allow patient connection. Practioners may also want to consider providing treatment in the home environment, where the person feels most comfortable and where many of these negative triggers are thus eliminated.

# SOCIAL STORIES—TEACCH AND PECS

A social story describes a situation, skill, or concept in terms of relevant social cues, perspectives, and common responses in a specifically defined style and format. The goal is to share accurate social information in a patient and reassuring manner that is easily understood by the audience. Social stories should affirm something that an individual does well. Although the goal should never be to change the individual's behavior, that individual's improved understanding of events and expectations may lead to more effective responses.

Although social stories were first developed for use with children with autism spectrum disorder (ASD), the approach has also been successful with children, adolescents, and adults with ASD and other social and communication delays and differences, as well as with individuals developing normally. Parents who use this process are familiar with it, and providing pictures and scenarios of the staff and environment that the person will personally experience is very helpful. Parents can make up these stories themselves. For many parents having the office create a social story and perhaps even a PowerPoint presentation that can be sent home prior to the first patient visit would ease much of the anxiety experienced at this first visit. Today it is even possible to have a short video clip on one's Web site that for some individuals may function even better. Having multiple alternatives satisfies the unique needs of persons with developmental disabilities.

Other techniques like TEACCH (Treatment and Education of Autistic and related Communication-handicapped CHildren), first developed by Mesibov and Schopler (Mesibov et al. 1994), are similar in that they provide cue cards for the individual with a precise breakdown of a procedure, thus enabling a person to understand each aspect of a procedure ahead of time. These visual schedules are utilized to make expectations clear and explicit, the intent being that communication does not require adult prompting. Morisaki et al. (2008) describe a case report where this procedure is used most effectively with a very difficult child with ASD.

PECS (Picture Exchange Communication System) is a similar form of augmentative/alternative communication system described by Bondy and Frost (1994) that also uses pictures as an aid in developing language skills and initiating communication for persons with developmental disabilities.

It is clear that many alternative communication strategies are currently in vogue. Being aware of the process being used by an individual can be helpful in adjusting one's approach to best align with that of the individual. For example, for a child who uses PECS it could be helpful to design a reinforcement sheet that uses this form of communication and not rely on the normal verbal or tangible reinforcements that may be used.

## SENSORY INTEGRATION

Although not unique to individuals with autism, sensory processing impairment is commonly seen in populations with developmental disabilities. Individuals with this impairment do not have the ability to integrate information across a variety of contexts (perception, attention, linguistic, and/or semantic) for higher-level meaning. The exact mechanism by which this occurs has a number of theories; however, all implicate atypical sensory processing as a core feature (Iarocci & McDonald 2006).

Individuals with hyposensitivity may feel little pain or enjoy sensations like strong tastes or intense pressure. Individuals with hypersensitivity may react more intensely to minimal touch, taste, or sound. Often combinations of these will occur in the same person.

Castillo Morales (personal communication) contends that by providing intense input for a sense that is being sought helps to allow an individual to tolerate further stimulation. For example, an individual who has a hyposensitivity to touch and does not like having his or her teeth brushed may do well with intense deep pressure. Applying firm pressure, first to the extremities; then to the forehead, eye area, cheeks, and chin; and only then proceeding intra-orally may result in the individual tolerating the brushing with greater ease.

- Touch is more tolerable when the child anticipates it.
- Many of these children find it easier to initiate hugging than to receive it.

- Firm, unmoving touch is better than light or moving touch.
- Light touch may be tolerable after firm unmoving touch.

It is important to determine the nature of what each individual feels most comfortable with. In some cases it will be vibration, followed by firm touch. No two individuals are the same. Most parents will be well aware of what comforts their child. However, parents may not recognize the relationship between daily oral care needs and these sensory impairments, and taking a few minutes to explain the impact and methods of intervening to the parent will help them to establish long-term healthy oral goals.

Sensory issues occur with people with other forms of disabilities as well. The same principle applies to these individuals. For example, applying firm vibratory pressure to a flexed foot in persons with cerebral palsy will often decrease uncontrollable movements of the head and body, allowing easier intra-oral stimulation, thus minimizing the need for protective support devices. Similarly, intra-oral massage can be used to decrease the gag reflex prior to brushing or oral exams. Shapiro et al. (2009) go further and show how the use of wraps or heavy leaded garments has been used with positive impact.

Having parents/caregivers complete a specific questionnaire highlighting these issues prior to an appointment may be very useful (Appendix 4.2.1).

# MUSIC THERAPY

Music therapy is a process in which a trained music therapist uses music and all of its facets—physical, emotional, mental, social, aesthetic, and spiritual—to help clients to improve or maintain their health. Music therapists primarily help clients improve their observable level of functioning and self-reported quality of life in various domains (e.g., cognitive functioning, motor skills, emotional and affective development, behavior and social skills) by using music experiences (e.g., singing, songwriting, listening to and discussing music, moving to music) to achieve measurable treatment goals and objectives. Music therapy, when paired with dental treatment, can be used not only to improve relaxation but also as a means to help in daily oral health regimes. Specific songs individualized for persons with disabilities can be used by all caregivers. It is not unusual for parents to sing some form of toothbrushing song while brushing their young children's teeth. This is a mere extension of what parents have known and done for centuries. Having favorite music on earphones or even using a singsong voice during procedures helps create an atmosphere of calm. For example, some evidence has shown that light classical music decreases nocturnal grinding in individuals with Down syndrome.

## CRANIOSACRAL THERAPY

During a craniosacral therapy session, the therapist places his or her hands on the patient, which allows him or her to tune into what is called the "craniosacral rhythm." The practitioner claims to gently work with the spinal column and skull and its cranial sutures. In this way, the restrictions of nerve passages are said to be eased, the movement of cerebrospinal fluid through the spinal cord is said to be optimized, and misaligned bones are said to be restored to their proper position. Craniosacral therapists use the therapy to treat mental stress, neck and back pain, temporomandibular joint disorders, and chronic pain. A session just prior to a dental appointment will often ease an individual's experience.

## EQUINE THERAPY

Equine therapy programs help teach people with disabilities companionship, responsibility, and leadership, as well as vocational and educational skills. Riding a horse provides a unique and often profound recreational or leisure activity for many people. Many programs around the world are dedicated to the various forms of horse riding or horse care and benefit even those who may not have a cognitive disability.

Equine therapy can be used for sensory integration and to help individuals develop meaningful and trusting relationships. Dentists in Argentina have used horses prior to dental treatment to help children receive care (IADH 2008). Horses are not judgmental and empower connection. The sometimes unpredictable nature of animals creates an environment in which individuals are able to confront fears and make adjustments to situations beyond their control.

## A CASE STUDY

Let us consider a 2-year-old with ASD. At the initial consultation appointment, the parents identify that he does not like having his mouth touched or his teeth brushed and they are also having difficulty with feeding. With the exception of the feeding issues, this would be quite common in any 2-year-old meeting the normal developmental milestones, and we would not hesitate to show the parents how to hold their child and initiate good oral health sanative behaviors. However, would holding and brushing or wiping with a cloth be the best method of care for a child with ASD? Castillo Morales has shown that children with sensitivity issues may benefit from desensitization prior to initiating any oral invasion. The two types of sensitivity would be pressure seeking and touch aversion. Most individuals with ASD are pressure seekers. In this case it is useful to first start with intense pressure therapy in an area away from the mouth, like the arms or legs, then gradually progress to the face area. One should start with the forehead, then move below the eyes, cheeks, and upper and lower lips, and end intra-orally from the anterior to the posterior. By initiating this desensitization the individual's trigger zones are inactivated, and he or she may better tolerate brushing, be less likely to gag, and also be more likely to have an easier time with eating. With those individuals who are touch aversive, gentle vibration of the feet and then the chest and back will often decrease the trigger zones and allow easier access.

This technique works at any age and when integrated with the repetitive tasking that is described above can mitigate the need for sedation or other advanced methods in a large percentage of individuals with developmental disabilities. This technique works with any individual with sensitivity issues and can be especially helpful for persons with cerebral palsy. In the latter, starting at the feet will in a short time help with uncontrollable movements and help settle individuals who would otherwise require some form of protective support to help immobilize them.

As Dr. Lyons says, desensitization is best learned as a daily stimulus and not as a semiannual event; thus it is imperative that the caregivers are instructed in the techniques used for desensitization and also that all involved in the caregiving have a common belief system as to the benefits.

Many individuals with disabilities make use of alternate methodologies for both health and educational care. It is useful to acknowledge their belief systems and utilize similar processes when working with these families. It is useful to mobilize what they already believe in.

## REFERENCES

Bondy AS, Frost LA. (1994). The Picture Exchange Communication System. *Focus on Autism and Other Developmental Disabilities* 9(3):1–19.

FlagHouse Inc. (2010). The philosophy & history of Snoezelen. Accessed August 2010 from http://www.flaghouse.com/philosophy_AL.asp.

Iarocci G, McDonald J. (2006). Sensory integration and the perceptual experience of persons with autism. *Journal of Autism and Developmental Disorders* 36(1):77–90.

International Association for Disability and Oral Health (IADH). (2008). 19th Congress of the IADH, October 29–31, Santos, Brazil. Conference proceedings.

Lehrner J, Marwinski G, Lehr S, Johren P, Deecke L. (2005). Ambient odors of orange and lavender reduce anxiety and improve mood in a dental office. *Physiology & Behavior* 86:92–95.

Mesibov GB, Schopler E, Hearsey KA. (1994). Structured teaching. In E. Schopler & G.B. Mesibov (Eds.), *Behavioral Issues in Autism* (pp. 195–207). New York: Plenum.

Miller WR, Rollnick S. (2002). *Motivational Interviewing*, 2nd ed. New York: Guildford Press.

Morisaki I, Ochiai TT, Akiyama S, Murakami J, Friedman CS. (2008). Behaviour guidance in dentistry for patients with autism spectrum disorder using a structured visual guide. *Journal of Disability and Oral Health* 9(3):136–140.

Robin O, Alaoui-Ismaili O, Dittmar A, Vernet-Maury E. (1999). Basic emotions evoked by eugenol odor differ according to dental experience: A neurovegetative analysis. *Chemical Senses* 24:327–335.

Shapiro M, Sgan-Cohen H, Parush S, Melmed R. (2009). Influence of adapted environment on the anxiety of medically treated children with developmental disability. *Journal of Pediatrics* 154:546–550.

Siegel DJ. (2010). *The Mindful Therapist: A Clinician's Guide to Mindsight and Neural Integration*. New York: W.W. Norton.

Thiemann KS, Goldstein H. (2001). Social stories, written text cues, and video feedback: Effects on social communication of children with autism. *Journal of Applied Behavior Analysis* 34(4):425–446.

# APPENDIX 4.2.1 (PLEASE NOTE: ALTHOUGH THE QUESTIONNAIRE BELOW IS INTENDED FOR CHILDREN, IT IS EASILY ADAPTED FOR ADULTS AS WELL.)

**PARENT/GUARDIAN—Questionnaire—Sensory/Educational Issues**

Child's Name: _____

Age: _____

Diagnosis: _____

_____

Medication: _____

_____

Communication:

Describe the primary form of communication:

      Verbal    Sign    PECS    TEACCH    Other

Describe the support system at school/workplace:

      Is there an educational assistant? Yes   No

      Is there a personalized program in place? Yes   No

      If yes, designed by whom? _____

      Describe: _____

      _____

What is the placement type? Circle one:

      Class integration

      Special education

      Special work environment

Socialization:

How does your child interact/react with peers or adults outside of home and school? Describe: _____

_____

What other supports or services have the family/child accessed? _____

_____

Is your child responsive to instructions? Yes   No

      If yes, please give examples. _____

      _____

To whom is your child most responsive? _____

_____

Can you make eye contact? Yes   No   If yes, for how long? _____

_____

Does your child have trouble separating at school, with doctors, or for haircuts? Yes   No

Does your child respond differently to men or women? Yes   No

      If yes, which produces a more positive response? _____

      _____

<u>Reinforcers</u> (i.e., favorite toys, items, activities, or treats that are used as rewards or to encourage positive behavior):
What is used at home? _____

What is used at school? _____

<u>Sensitivities:</u>
Is your child sensitive to any of the following? Circle those that apply and add any we have missed.

       Smell—office, perfume, cologne
       Sounds—music, drill, phones, voices, clock
       Sight—lights, overhead arm, mirrors, shiny tools
       Positions—chair height and tilt, being "still," lying flat
       Proximity—people, water, light, x-ray machine
       Touch/temp—gloves, air, gauze, water, suction, room and water
          temperature, toothbrushing, feeding
       Texture—toothpaste, gauze, cotton, metal
       Pressure—seeking or aversion
       Taste—gloves, toothpaste, fluoride

How does your child indicate this sensitivity? _____

How have you responded to these sensitivities in the past? _____

How has this method worked? _____

<u>Diet:</u>
Foods preferences—list: _____

Food aversions/dislikes—list:_____

<u>Summary:</u>
What are your goals for your child in our office? _____

What are your expectations for your child?_____

What would be your idea of success? _____

What are you prepared to do in order to accomplish this goal? _____

# Section 3: Aging population supports

## Paul S. Farsai, DMD, MPH and Joseph M. Calabrese, DMD, FACD

In 2008, an estimated 12% of non-institutionalized, male or female, all ages, all races, regardless of ethnicity, with all education levels in the United States (thirty-six million out of three hundred million people) reported a disability (Cornell University 2008; Waldman et al. 2010). This percentage doubles to 26% when we consider the 65–74 age group and increases to over 51% when we take into account those individuals aged 75 and over. When treating older adults it is important to understand that the dental issues relevant to the healthy aging population are different than for those who are aging with disabilities (Waldman & Perlman 1997).

## OLDER ADULTS WITH DISABILITIES

Dental treatment for adults living with disabilities may be provided in hospitals, long-term care facilities, skilled nursing facilities, group homes, private practice, or community health centers. It typically involves modifying the dental examination and the required dental treatment due to the patient's disability and age-related conditions and symptoms.

Dental care for older patients with developmental disorders often involves consulting with one or more members of the patient's health care team. This effort may include but not be limited to coordinating dental treatment with other care providers, accommodating a person with the aid of the caregivers, adapting the treatment procedure, communicating

*Treating the Dental Patient with a Developmental Disorder*, First Edition.
Edited by Karen A. Raposa and Steven P. Perlman.
© 2012 John Wiley & Sons, Inc. Published 2012 by John Wiley & Sons, Inc.

through an interpreter, or customizing treatment plans with the patient's potential for future oral health problems in mind.

Oral diseases for older individuals with developmental disabilities do not differ from those of older individuals without disabilities. However, various factors related to an aging individual's disability may make it more difficult to assess, prevent, and treat dental disease. For instance, someone suffering from arthritis can have difficulty grasping a toothbrush, while someone with a cognitive disorder as well as arthritis may have difficulty recognizing the functionality of the toothbrush he or she is having difficulty grasping. Treatment may also differ because the disease is typically addressed at a later stage due to infrequent checkups, avoidance, lack of resources, inability to articulate that a problem exists, or other common geriatric-related access to care issues. Often the care must be adapted to the individual's physical and cognitive impairments.

Therefore, just as dental providers make adjustments to the treatment for elderly patients, it is envisioned that the dental care for those individuals with disabilities shall require similar modifications. We will discuss and elaborate upon many of these modifications in this chapter.

While reading through this section we ask that you consider two viewpoints simultaneously. One view is the (primary) preventive aspect of dentistry, which considers all the harmful possibilities with foresight for diseases or conditions and prophylactically applies the preventive regimens to those oral conditions so they are never manifested or, if they are, it is with a much lower incidence rate. The second approach is the more prevalent therapeutic or rehabilitative aspect of dentistry (secondary prevention). This approach is taken once the disease or condition is encountered and is typically treated rapidly. This is the approach where we have typically spent most of our time and efforts in dentistry.

The more experience one gains treating the dental needs of older adults with special needs, the more one understands that each person is different with respect to the manifestation of these conditions. In certain situations preventive and therapeutic approaches when applied collectively can significantly improve the patient's oral experience. The decision to use one approach over another, or both, is a function of what the oral health status is at the time of the examination.

The idea is to illicit a model or thought process for the practitioner where treating as well as preventing disease becomes the rule when a patient presents to the dentist. If the patient presents with no disease—an approach of "do more now to *prevent* in order to do less treatment later" is recommended.

## COMMON CHANGES IN THE ORAL CAVITY ENCOUNTERED IN OLDER ADULTS WITH DISABILITIES

Certain oral conditions appear more often in persons with specific disabilities due in part because of the disability but also because of the behavior patterns that go hand in hand with the actual disability. For example, in persons with intellectual disabilities (such as Down syndrome), there is an altered eruption pattern of teeth (Pilcher 1998). The altered eruption pattern is oftentimes due to overretained primary teeth or even the malformation of an individual's teeth (atypical shape and anatomy of teeth).

The delayed eruption patterns tend to lead to malocclusion if left untreated. In this population if the issue is not addressed in adolescence, then an exacerbated oral condition will be encountered later on in life with respect to caries rate, caries risk, infection, and subsequent periodontal disease sequelae because of the untreated oral condition(s).

- *Fractured teeth* are commonly seen in the anterior region of individuals with neurodevelopmental disabilities. For older individuals with these types of disabilities, the prevalence rate is higher because these teeth have been repeatedly restored. In most cases the size of the restorations and/or the type of restorative work is more involved. This is due to several physical factors such as poor ambulatory skills and depletion of motor skills, as well as seizure disorders. However, any tooth in an individual with developmental disabilities that had been previously restored will also be at risk for more frequent fractures. This is especially true in an elderly cohort where older generations of restorative materials were used or other disease patterns were once addressed.
- *Xerostomia* is a common and often overlooked oral health problem. Once considered an inevitable consequence of aging, it is now known that saliva production remains essentially unchanged in healthy elders (Närhi 1994; Locker 1993). However, the secretion of the saliva may be indirectly dependent on the systemic health of a person, as well as the number and type of medications that the person is taking. Medications used to treat high blood pressure, heart disease, diabetes, allergies, depression, and many other conditions have been found to cause xerostomia (Ship et al. 2002; Närhi et al. 1999). Saliva helps to maintain a healthy oral environment by limiting bacteria, remineralizing teeth, lubricating tissues, and enhancing taste sensation (Dodds et al. 2005).

  Change in salivary flow may impair complete or full denture retention and increase oral trauma from a removable prosthesis. Diminished salivary flow is associated with increased burning/soreness of the oral tissues; difficulty chewing, speaking, and swallowing; and oral infections, all of which can adversely affect food selection and dietary compliance.

  With the extensive benefits of salivary production known to dental care providers, one can only postulate how an altered salivary flow may contribute to behavioral issues with patients who have limited communication skills, are aging, and are developing increasing dental problems (Fisher & Kettl 2005). As the individual with a developmental disability ages, the problems in fact do not necessarily become easier to treat. Hyposalivation can present difficult challenges to both the afflicted patient and the dental practitioner.

Dry mouth can further contribute to the accumulation of debris around teeth, which can lead to advanced stages of dental caries, periodontal disease, or consequent tooth loss.

- *Caries* is not uncommon in the aging population. This process typically occurs when the food debris and bacteria are not adequately removed from the teeth. What exacerbates this process in the elderly in addition to xerostomia is the fact that manual dexterity is also decreased for home care. The addition of inadequate home care along with the daily management of an intellectual or developmental disability will clearly influence the caries rate in the negative direction. As one ages, the difficulty in mastication or the ease of chewing becomes a factor in food selection as well. Individuals tend to select foods that are easier to prepare but oftentimes tend to be high in sugar and carbohydrates, which can also make one more susceptible to caries if the teeth are not cleaned appropriately.

- *Root caries* becomes a problem when attachment loss and the subsequent gingival recession cause the exposure of the more porous cementum. This increase of the less mineralized tooth surface to the harmful effects of the decay process makes root caries another problem. Oral hygiene measures and adaptive aids to decrease the food accumulation on teeth and root surfaces are instrumental in the prevention of root caries. Because of root structure anatomy and the proximity of nerve tissue to the surface of the root, the root decay can spread much more rapidly to the nerve of the tooth, leading to the need for root canal therapy. The type and ease of use of the dental restorative material to address the root cavity preparation is also a consideration for the elderly person with an intellectual or developmental disability. Stressing or inconveniencing an elderly person for a repeated dental procedure has to be taken into account. As described earlier in this chapter, the approach of prevention first in order to minimize subsequent procedures is of utmost importance.

- *Gingivitis* and *periodontitis* are also commonly observed in the geriatric individual with intellectual or developmental disability. As described earlier in the caries sections, the inadequate removal of food and bacteria from the teeth often leads to inflammatory gingival and periodontal disease processes. Oral hygiene protocols such as brushing, flossing, and rinsing with mouthwashes can help arrest or reverse the gingival problems. The real concern is following a supervised regimen of oral hygiene care that is often nonexistent in the life of an older individual with an intellectual or developmental disability. Such high-level supervised care is difficult to find and extremely costly. Caretakers are usually more concerned with other activities of daily living than with oral hygiene. Similarly, the more advanced therapies for periodontal disease imply that the individual with a disability is able to tolerate a surgical appointment without the benefit of understanding what the procedure entails. This may not always be the case. An additional factor to consider is the provider's comfort level in performing an invasive procedure on a patient who may not be physically or behaviorally tolerant of that level of care in a dental chair.

- *Missing teeth* (and tooth loss) can be a very upsetting trial in one's life, particularly if the missing teeth are not replaced. The three most common causes of tooth loss are advanced tooth decay; advanced periodontal disease; and trauma from falls, seizures, or accidents. Many options are available today for patients seeking treatment to replace their missing teeth. However, the cost, the duration of treatment, and the provider's ability to perform these procedures (sometimes in a non-traditional environment or with major modifications) make replacing missing teeth a difficult process in an individual with intellectual or developmental disabilities.

- *Tooth replacement* (dental prosthesis) is done to fill the spaces left by missing teeth so the patient is restored to some means of original form and function. The need to restore function and aesthetic value can play an important role to help improve any individual's quality of life. Appropriate treatment options for an older individual with a disability will depend on many factors. These include the costs, the time required to do the procedure, and the patient's tolerance during the appointment(s). Other factors include number of visits required to complete the procedure and skill level of the involved in managing the individual with the disability.

- *Bad breath* (halitosis) is caused by a number of factors. It is often due to upper respiratory conditions caused by excessive mucous buildup, infections, or even poor digestion. However, halitosis can very easily originate in the oral cavity due to inadequate oral hygiene, large cavities, or even advanced periodontitis.

- *Food pocketing* (pouching) is a condition where individuals who are unable to chew or swallow for any of the above-mentioned reasons accumulate their food between their cheeks/lips and their soft tissues. Many medications are coated with sugar to help patients swallow, and pouching of food debris and medications not only results in significant dental decay and medical consequences but also leads to malnutrition.

- *Regurgitation* (rumination) is a characteristic seen in many individuals with intellectual disabilities. With this condition, individuals swallow their food and then regurgitate it with the stomach fluids/acids, leading to severe indigestion and malnutrition. Oftentimes in patients who have excessive drooling of saliva, dental professionals will need to consider the oral hygiene problems with pouching and frequency of food intake prior to the dental appointments to minimize regurgitation as well.

- *Oral cancer* is predominantly caused by risk factors such as smoking and alcohol abuse; more recently, evidence has shown that the human papilloma virus (HPV) is becoming one of the leading causes of oral cancer (CDC 2004; Western Dental Services 2011). Although there is no significant data available relating oral cancer to adults with disabilities, we do know that individuals with disabilities are living longer and more meaningful lives and should be evaluated regularly for any suspicious oral lesions.

# WHAT TO LOOK FOR IN DENTAL TREATMENT FOR OLDER ADULTS WITH DISABILITIES

Following a comprehensive clinical examination, the dentist will present treatment options to the patient and/or caregiver or family member.

In the general population, older adults are keeping their natural teeth longer than ever before (Cornell University 2008). Although dental statistics for aging individuals with disabilities are not well documented, it would not be surprising to see a higher frequency of advanced and neglected dental problems in this older population with disabilities.

The dental treatment plan should be formulated according to accepted dental practice, yet it should also allow for certain modifications to take place based on consideration for some basic factors such as:

- Addressing the patient's immediate pain or infection.
- Patient's mental status—the level of disability, understanding and communication, psychological and social needs.
- The effects of the current oral condition on the quality of life.
- Physical impairments.
- Performing as much treatment as possible while taking into account the patient capacity for care and management.
- Financial considerations .
- A "prevention" modality for current and future dental care.

# RECOMMENDATIONS FOR APPROPRIATE ORAL HYGIENE

- *Toothbrushing*—toothbrushes can be modified to enable aging patients with physical and intellectual disabilities to brush their own teeth and decrease the incidence of pouching (see the information on adaptive aids). Certain powered (rotary) toothbrushes may improve patient compliance as well. For individuals who are unable to perform this task independently because of a physical disability, there are several simple, homemade adaptive methods available. By cutting two slices on opposing sides of a tennis ball or a racquetball and inserting the handle of a toothbrush through the two perforations, the older patient is allowed to first of all grasp and also gain a more firm grip for toothbrushing. Other materials such as pipe insulation, athletic tape, or even cutoff rubber bicycle grips can be creatively used to provide an adaptation for better manual dexterity as with the tennis ball grip described above.

Similarly, if the patient is combative and will not allow for the task of toothbrushing, a washcloth dampened with mouthwash can be the next best option to wipe the teeth clean from debris.

- Use of *fluoride toothpaste* or *gel* has been extensively shown in dental studies to maximize the effects of caries reduction regimens and to increase the longevity of restorative dental procedures in the aging population with intellectual and developmental disabilities. A good oral health promotion and disease prevention regimen always consists of some combination of fluoride therapy whether in toothpaste, gel, or an oral rinse. This regimen is even more important for individuals who have limited intellectual capacity for brushing, have behavioral or management constraints, or have developmental disabilities that render them more susceptible to dental problems.

- *Flossing* should be part of a daily routine; however, it may be difficult for individuals with certain intellectual or physical disabilities to perform such tasks. A second person who is more familiar with and trusted by the patient as well as adequately trained may be required to assist with flossing. Flossing with floss holders (or, if tolerated, using power flossers) can help older patients with manual dexterity issues and decrease dependence on others for their oral health and prevention needs.

- *Mouthwashes* and toothpastes (and gels) are beneficial in managing dental decay as well as gingivitis and subsequent risk for periodontal disease. It is important to recognize that today there are various ingredients in these products. Dentists should understand the function of these ingredients in order to better match these products with the needs of the older patients with disabilities. Over-the-counter (OTC) oral rinses and toothpastes now contain anti-bacterial agents, fluoride (in various derivatives), and tooth-whitening agents. For those patients suffering from xerostomia, nonalcoholic rinses are available, and for those requiring a higher level of prevention, prescription-strength anti-bacterial agents with chlorhexidine are available in rinses. For those who need to address chronic nondental-related halitosis with a more pleasant taste, some OTC rinses contain natural sweeteners such as xylitol instead of sugar. This can make patients more compliant with their use of OTC rinses. Triclosan is an active anti-fungal and anti-bacterial agent that is found in certain OTC toothpaste/gels.

Anti-bacterial rinses are most effective when used in conjunction with and immediately following a dental prophylaxis. However, it is recommended for special needs patients to use a prescription mouthwash with the active ingredient chlorhexidine or at the least an OTC anti-bacterial rinse. Mouthwashes should be swished and spit out (never swallowed); patients who might swallow a rinse could benefit from its application with a toothbrush or cotton swab rather than swishing with a larger volume of mouth rinse.

- *Dietary counseling* is necessary for long-term prevention of dental disease, weight management, and overall health (Henshaw & Calabrese 2001). The relationships among oral health, adequate nutrition, and dietary intake needed for physiologic function are multifaceted (Walls et al. 2000; Soini et al. 2003). This is especially significant in aging individuals with developmental disorders who have a compromised health status or have difficulty chewing or swallowing.
- *Dental recall*—while most people visit their dentist and hygienist bi-annually, special needs adults should be scheduled in accordance with their needs and abilities. For the older individuals with developmental disabilities, this may mean more frequent visits to the dental office. Because oral hygiene practices are not always as optimal in the aging population with developmental disabilities, dental diseases become more prevalent in this population. In severe cases where dental disease is more prevalent, recall intervals as well as restorative work may need to be as often as every 2 or 3 months. After the initial phase of treatment is completed and oral disease has been eliminated, then the visits can be adjusted to more routine intervals of every 3, 4, or 6 months if oral health improvement is observed.

## ISSUES TO CONSIDER WHEN SELECTING A DENTIST

Some important issues to consider when selecting a dentist for the care of an aging individual with disabilities should include:

- *Transportation*—is the dental office/health center easily accessible by motor vehicle? Is public transportation available to and from the office? Is it in a convenient location?
- *Building (physical structure and environment)*—can the parking lot accommodate a chair-van? Is there a ramp available to facilitate transport of a person in a wheelchair or a walker? Are the treatment rooms and restrooms wheelchair accessible? Are the walkways wide enough to accommodate wheelchairs, walkers, or caregivers supporting immobile patients?
- *Training/education/experience*—does the dental professional (dentist or hygienist) provide special care dentistry specifically for aging patients? Has he or she had training in special care dentistry? If needed, can treatment be rendered in a hospital setting? Does the dental care provider feel comfortable in providing care for special needs patients? Are the hours convenient?
- *Treatment goals*—appropriate patient treatment goals include stabilizing and improving the oral condition of the patient. Stabilization of the oral condition keeps individuals who have not received routine care or have received poor or inappropriate care free of acute disease. In no way should the previous statement be conceived as a negative comment toward a

dental team member who provided prior care for an aging individual with developmental disabilities; however, it is reflective of the common understanding and acceptance in the dental community of the need for more clinical and behavioral management training for dental team members. Oftentimes even with the best of intentions a dental care provider is unable to perform his or her best service because of a lack of the management skills or the background knowledge on aging and developmental disabilities to take care of an individual with such disabilities.

Most of the acute oral conditions that are commonly seen in older adults as well as in individuals who have physical, intellectual, or developmental disabilities have been discussed in this section. However, a clinical examination may reveal other oral conditions that will need appropriate or even immediate care. These conditions common in older individuals with developmental disabilities are candidiasis, moniliasis, lichen planus, chronic ulcerations, fistulas, and stomatitis. With the onset of some more recent observations of osteonecrosis of the jaw (ONJ) due to bone cancer therapy and the use of bis-phosphonates, clinicians must be even more vigilant in their clinical assessments of older adults with developmental disabilities. This is the reason why a comprehensive clinical exam cannot be overemphasized.

Once the patient is stabilized from acute disease in as many appointments as is necessary, the next phase of therapy will be the restoration of the patient's teeth and missing spaces in order to address the oral health and function of the aging patient. The completion of this phase of therapy is followed by an appropriate individualized, risk-based preventative maintenance schedule designed to oversee the patient's reestablished oral health.

## STEPS TO TAKE

What steps should older adults with disabilities and their caretakers take to assist in the prevention and maintenance of the oral cavity?

Given the patient's level of impairment or disability, the first step in obtaining compliance with oral hygiene recommendations is by promoting the patient's involvement through education and demonstration. This level of involvement maximizes the patient's acceptance of his or her oral condition and partially promotes independence with respect to oral health. If the patient is unable to participate in the educational/instructional process, the caregiver is encouraged to assume this responsibility for the patient.

Educating family members or other caregivers is also critical for ensuring appropriate and regular supervision of daily oral hygiene. Caregivers should monitor the patient's oral care daily and provide oral care assistance when the patient is unable to do so. Specifically, the caregiver or family member's supervision of the aging individual with developmental disabilities should include a specific routine of oral care, preferably around the same time each day. This supervision may include removing any appliance(s) prior to brushing and rinsing, physically supporting or aiding the patient for routine daily toothbrushing, visually inspecting the quality of oral hygiene performance, and encouraging the individual during and after the activity. More often than not the family member or caregiver may need to clean any appliance(s) for the patient. The most important factor, however, is making the supervised routine a daily activity.

Such supervised care can be facilitated with proper positioning of the aging patient with the aid of pillows, beanbags, airbags, and smaller/larger chairs.

Certain "adaptive aids" such as large-sized toothbrush handles or, as mentioned earlier, use of a tennis ball or racquetball may improve the manual dexterity and physical manipulation of a toothbrush. Other useful and appropriate material used in the oral health care of an aging individual with physical disabilities and developmental disorders may include the use of powered (rotary) toothbrushes, anti-microbial and fluoridated mouth rinses, and oral lubricants that resolve oral discomfort associated with the gum tissues.

Depending on where the individual with the disability resides (home, nursing home, or other long-term care facility), the primary caregiver can be a family member, nurse's aid, nurse practitioner, and/or other persons. If oral hygiene care is seen as a shared responsibility, then obtaining assistance to provide basic oral hygiene for the patient may be helpful in decreasing the level of responsibility for the primary caregiver. This could provide an additional monitoring system for the patient's oral hygiene routine as well.

## BARRIERS TO TREATMENT

Aside from the oral health care supports needed by many individuals with disabilities, there are other significant barriers that prevent access to proper oral health care.

- *Insufficient numbers of dental health providers*—clinicians who are often charged with providing the oral health care for adults living with intellectual and developmental disabilities are cognizant of the necessity to address the oral health care needs of these individuals. Many times these individuals can be treated by the small number of clinicians that have formal training in geriatric dental medicine. However, more often than not these patients are referred back to the pediatric dentist for treatment. The reality that needs to be recognized by the profession and collectively addressed in the coming years is that individuals are living longer and they are doing so with more chronic diseases. Individuals with developmental and intellectual disabilities are living longer with a significantly higher level of dependence on others. Their age-related and physiologic changes need to be addressed by providers who understand all of their disabilities. Informing those oral health providers by means of the information in this book is a way to begin the process of training current and future oral health providers.

Most dentists already treat older adults with certain physical impairments and medical conditions. As health care improves and many of the once acute and advanced conditions become chronic or manageable conditions, these patients will continue to grow in number and seek care from traditional private or community-based services. At the same time, individuals who have long-term disabilities continue to live longer because of improvements in the management of their conditions through various social and medical services.

Greater numbers of patients with mental retardation and related intellectual and developmental disabilities require oral health care that accommodates their impairments, including physical and behavioral support during the dental treatment.

- *Informed consent and treatment decisions*—a major determining factor in providing any type of treatment accommodation for the patient with a disability is the need to obtain informed consent for treatment. Most individuals with intellectual disabilities have a legal guardian, health care proxy, or caretaker that is authorized to consent to the proposed treatment. However, as in the case of many older individuals with intellectual or developmental disabilities, a caregiver may not necessarily be the appointed health care proxy or the individual authorized to make dental care decisions and may be an individual who is not very well aware of or concerned with the dental needs of his or her loved one. It is integral for the oral health provider to communicate the necessity of oral health to all involved parties including the family, health care proxy, caregivers, and legal guardians. It is then highly recommended that the immediate family member or health care proxy of the aging individual with a developmental disability becomes the "supervisor" of the oral health care regimens conducted by the caregivers.

  The person who provides consent also needs to understand that in certain instances, such as individuals with severe disabilities, it is neither possible nor feasible to render care, as doing so may endanger or have no effect on the patient's health or quality of life.

  The determination of providing care or no care by the health professional is typically a function of several factors such as a thorough understanding of the patient's condition, the level of comfort and training of the health professional, and the availability of financial resources. Many times, this decision is the greatest challenge that the treating clinician will face regarding treatment.

- *Inadequate financial coverage*—another barrier that clearly prevents properly addressing the dental needs of aging individuals with developmental disorders is the poor reimbursement for dental services. The lack of adequate financial coverage for an adult with developmental disorders may dictate certain compromises in the dental treatment plan or even denial of dental services.

Medicare is the largest federally funded health care system in the United States for older adults, yet it does not include a specific dental component.

Medicaid, which is a needs-based health and social services program, can be a source of payment for dental services, but not all state Medicaid plans offer dental care coverage for adults (i.e., over age 18 or in certain states over age 21). Typically dental coverage is limited and varies among states. In times of economic hardship and budgetary constraints, local and federal governments typically tend to cut the dental benefits of Medicaid programs for adults. Fortunately, there are also individual states that have maintained the adult dental benefits for those with intellectual and developmental disabilities during the same economic and budgetary downfall periods. An additional financial barrier for older adults with developmental disabilities is that a majority of dentists in most states are not Medicaid providers. Thus the scope of dental services can be even more limited depending on the number of Medicaid providers in the patient's state of residence.

Another variable that further complicates issues for Medicaid coverage in many states is the eligibility restrictions for adults due to the level of disability. In other words, adults who may have a "lower" yet still significant level of disability (mild to moderate level of disability) may not be eligible for Medicaid.

Sometimes reimbursement, although at a lower level, is available for certain types of dental care through Medicaid waiver programs, grants through local and state dental societies/associations, or through certain guidelines with developmental disabilities councils. State dental societies are good resources to receive more information about these programs.

State-run agencies such as public health clinics and community health centers can also serve as resources for obtaining proper access to oral health care. Many aging individuals with disabilities have access to social workers, support coordinators, or caseworkers that may be able to assist in obtaining full or partial funding for specific dental services. Most important, the issue of finding a skilled dental practitioner, cognizant in the ways and methods of treating older adults with disabilities, is still the fundamental concern.

# REFERENCES

Centers for Disease Control. (2004). Health consequences of smoking: A report of the Surgeon General. U.S. Department of Health and Human Services.

Cormier PP. (1982). Who is handicapped: The patient or the provider? *Journal of Dental Education* 46(3):166–169.

Cornell University. (2008). Disability status report: United States. Accessed August 17 and 31, 2010, from www.ilr.cornell.edu/edi/disabilitystatistics/reports/acs.cfm?statistic=1.

Dodds M, Johnson D, Yeh C. (2005). Health benefits of saliva: A review. *Journal of Dentistry* 33(3):223–233.

Fisher K, Kettl P. (2005). Aging with mental retardation—increasing population of older adults with MR require health interventions and prevention strategies. *Geriatrics* 60(4):26–29.

Henshaw MM, Calabrese JM. (2001). Oral health and nutrition in the elderly. *Nutrition in Clinical Care* 4(1):34–42.

Krahn GL, Hammond L, Turner A. (2006). A cascade of disparities: Health and health care access for people with intellectual disabilities. *Mental Retardation and Developmental Disabilities Research Reviews* 12(1):70–82.

Locker D. (1993). Subjective reports of oral dryness in an older adult population. *Community Dentistry and Oral Epidemiology* 21(3):165–168.

Närhi T. (1994). Prevalence of subjective feelings of dry mouth in the elderly. *Journal of Dental Research* 73(1):20–25.

Närhi TO, Meurman JH, Ainamo A. (1999). Xerostomia and hyposalivation: Causes, consequences and treatment in the elderly. *Drugs and Aging* 15(2):103–116.

Perlman SP. (2000). Helping Special Olympics athletes sport good smiles: An effort to reach out to people with special needs. *Dental Clinics of North America* 44(1):221–229.

Pilcher ES. (1998). Dental care for the patient with Down syndrome. *Down Syndrome Research and Practice* 5(3):111–116.

Ship JA, Pillemer SR, Baum BJ. (2002). Xerostomia and the geriatric patient. *Journal of the American Geriatrics Society* 50(3):535–543.

Soini H, Routasalo P, Sirkka L, et al. (2003). Oral and nutritional status in frail elderly. *Special Care in Dentistry* 23(6):209–215.

Waldman HB, Perlman SP. (1997). Children with disabilities are aging out of care. *Journal of Dentistry for Children* 64(6):385–390.

Waldman HB, Perlman SP, Rader R. (2010). Guest editorial: The transition of children with disabilities to adulthood—what about dental care? *Journal of the American Dental Association* 141:937–938.

Waldman HB, Perlman SP, Swerdloff M. (1998). What if dentists did not treat people with disabilities? *Journal of Dentistry for Children* 65:96–101.

Walls A, Steele J, Sheinham A, et al. (2000). Oral health and nutrition in older people. *Journal of Public Health Dentistry* 60(4):304–307.

Western Dental Services, Inc. (2011). Recognizing the symptoms of oral cancer. Accessed May 20, 2011, from http://www.disabled-world.com/health/cancer/oral-cancer.php.

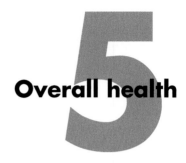

# Overall health

## Matthew Holder, MD, MBA and Henry Hood, DMD

## OVERVIEW

In treating patients with developmental disorders, dental practitioners find themselves facing unique challenges that are not common in other patient populations. Because patients with developmental disorders are more reliant upon the system of care that surrounds them, they suffer greater health consequences when that system of care breaks down. In order to decrease the likelihood of health system failure, health professionals from all disciplines need a more holistic view of the patient and of patient care. This can be achieved through greater interdisciplinary understanding and communication. Dentists who have a greater neurobiological understanding of the whole patient will be more effective members and leaders of the health care team upon which their patients rely.

## TERMINOLOGY

For clinicians first beginning to work with this patient population, one of the most immediate challenges is understanding the terminology used in different professional, advocacy, and legal circles that refers, often imprecisely, to the same (or nearly the same) population.

*Treating the Dental Patient with a Developmental Disorder*, First Edition.
Edited by Karen A. Raposa and Steven P. Perlman.
© 2012 John Wiley & Sons, Inc. Published 2012 by John Wiley & Sons, Inc.

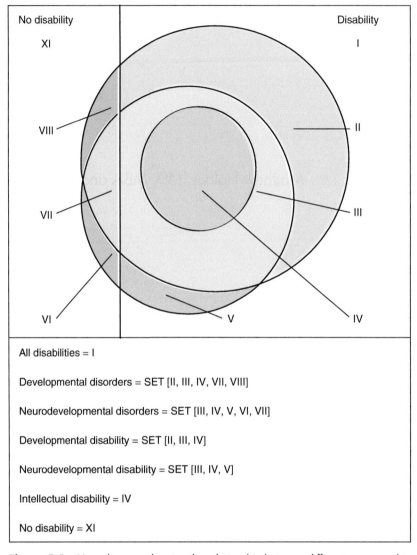

**Figure 5.1** Venn diagram showing the relationship between different terms used to describe this patient population.

Two terms that should not be used when describing this population are "mental retardation" and "cognitive impairment." "Mental retardation" is an outdated term that is increasingly being viewed as offensive to people within the disability community. The term "mental retardation" has been effectively replaced with the synonymous term "intellectual disability" (ID) (Schalock et al. 2007).

"Cognitive impairment" is often mistakenly used as a synonym for "intellectual disability." Though functionally the adult patient with cognitive impairment and the adult patient with ID may be indistinguishable, cognitive impairment is a much more broad term that can refer to both temporary and permanent intellectual states and may include an onset of symptoms during either childhood or adulthood. As an example, cognitive impairment could refer to a temporary state of drug-induced delirium in a 70-year-old patient or a permanent state of ID caused by trisomy 21.

In the United States, there are five widely used terms that often refer to the same population: "intellectual disability," "neurodevelopmental disability," "neurodevelopmental disorder," "developmental disability," and "developmental disorder." Though there is significant overlap among these five terms, it is important to appreciate the relationships and the differences among them. Figure 5.1 shows the relationships among these terms. In order to better understand this, consider that the entire population is divided into two segments, those who are disabled and those who are not disabled. Though what factors determine "disability" can often be vague, for purposes of this illustration consider that there are two groups of people and that the difference between these two groups is easily demarcated by a line.

The most broad term is "developmental disorder." A natural subset of people with developmental disorders are those whose disorders have led to a disability, thus they are people with a developmental disability. Closely overlapping the set of people with developmental disorders is the set of people with neurodevelopmental disorders. The reason that the latter is not a perfect subset of the former has to do with the underlying vocational fields that define the terms. "Developmental disability" and thus "developmental disorder," by extension, are often sociologically or legally defined terms, whereas "neurodevelopmental disorder" and thus "neurodevelopmental disability," by extension, are biologically defined terms. A natural subset of neurodevelopemental disorder is neurodevelopmental disability, that is, neurodevelopmental disorders that have resulted in disability. Finally, found within all of the previous sets mentioned is the set of people with ID.

## Intellectual disability

Intellectual disability is characterized by significant limitations in both intellectual functioning and adaptive behavior as expressed in conceptual, social, and practical skills. This disability originates before age 18 (Schalock et al. 2010). It is a common symptom of multiple developmental and neurodevelopmental disorders.

## Neurodevelopmental disability

Neurodevelopmental disabilities are disabilities that can be attributed to neurodevelopmental disorders. Some neurodevelopmental disabilities are well defined and others are not. Intellectual disability is one type of neurodevelopmental disability. Autism (that is severe enough to be recognized as a disability) could be construed as a neurodevelopmental disability. Cerebral palsy in many cases could be considered a neurodevelopmental disability as well. Neurodevelopmental disability overlaps considerably, by definition, with developmental disability.

## Neurodevelopmental disorder

A neurodevelopmental disorder is a genetic or acquired biological process, occurring before adulthood, that disrupts one or more of the expected functions of the brain, resulting in one or more common complications. Such complications include: (1) intellectual disability, (2) neuromotor dysfunction, (3) sensory impairment, (4) seizure disorder, and (5) abnormal behavior. Neurodevelopmental disorders, depending upon their etiology, can be associated with various syndrome-specific conditions. Both the common complications and syndrome-specific conditions can, and often do, lead to secondary health consequences. These characteristics of neurodevelopmental disorders will be discussed further in this chapter (Rader 2007).

## Developmental disability

Developmental disability is a socio-legal construct. Because its definitional roots are not biologically based, the definition can vary from state to state. Under most circumstances, neurodevelopmental disability would be considered a subset of developmental disability; however, because both definitions can be ambiguous as to the age at onset of symptoms, it is possible for some patients to be considered to have a neurodevelopmental disability while not having a developmental disability. Though the definition of developmental disability can vary, a typical definition would include but is not limited to people who have an ID, autism, cerebral palsy, a severe seizure disorder, or a severe head injury that occurs before the age of 18.

Under federal law, developmental disability means a severe, chronic disability of an individual that (1) is attributable to a mental or physical impairment or combination of mental and physical impairments; (2) is manifested before the age of 22; (3) is likely to continue indefinitely; (4) results in substantial functional limitations in three or more of the following areas of major life activity: self-care, receptive and expressive language, learning, mobility, self-direction, capacity for independent living, economic self-sufficiency; and (5) reflects the individual's need for services, supports, or other forms of assistance that are of lifelong or extended duration and are individually planned and coordinated (Developmental Disabilities Assistance and Bill of Rights Act of 2000).

## Developmental disorder

A developmental disorder is the biological cause of the underlying developmental disability. Most neurodevelopmental disorders, such as Down syndrome, fragile X syndrome, and fetal alcohol syndrome, are also considered developmental disorders. Developmental disorders may also encompass other disorders of nonneurologic origin such as muscular dystrophy.

# COMMON CHARACTERISTICS

In general, regardless of the terminology used to describe this patient population, there are common biological characteristics that will affect patient care. Though people with purely physical disabilities may require special accommodations, it is the patients with neurodevelopmental disorders that tend to present the greatest challenge for the dental practitioner. Understanding the characteristics of these patients and appropriately adjusting the clinical approach to the patient based on these common characteristics will ensure the greatest chance of clinical success.

## Etiology

No matter how the patient presents, it is important to remember that all disabilities have a cause. Very often patients will arrive at the clinic with the "diagnosis" of intellectual disability, with no other explanation. As clinicians it is important to attempt to ascertain the underlying cause of the ID. There are potentially thousands of causes of intellectual disability that exist. Though many causes are still unknown, as the state of science has evolved, more and more causes of ID are being described. Determining etiology is important because etiology can affect prognosis and determine specific preventive health measures that can be taken. Intellectual disability caused by Down syndrome, for example, leads the clinician to a much different clinical picture than ID due to lead toxicity. Knowing the etiology can greatly affect preventive health measures and, just as importantly, can be very powerful information for family members. Such information will not only guide the care of the patient; if it is an inherited disorder it may also have a significant effect on future family planning (Box 5.1).

In order to help discover etiologies, dentists should familiarize themselves with some of the more common morphologic features of the head and neck of the more recognizable syndromes. Though Down syndrome can be recognized by most clinicians, many other syndromes such as fragile X, Prader-Willi, Angelman, Williams, fetal alcohol, Cornelia de Lange, Turner, and Sturge-Weber have distinctive physical features that can be recognized by the dentist. If a dentist suspects that a patient may have a previously undiagnosed syndrome, he or she should not hesitate to refer the patient to a geneticist for further evaluation. Because of the rapidly advancing field of genetics, even if the patient had a negative genetic evaluation in the past, if that evaluation is more than 10 years old, the patient may benefit from another evaluation.

---

**Box 5.1**   Family perspective on the value of a diagnosis.

I can say that, for us, it really was helpful to get (our child's) diagnosis. When preliminary testing did not provide answers, they told us that a diagnosis probably would not affect the treatment approach and they did not see much reason to look further. They diagnosed (our child) with cerebral palsy and mental retardation; we were fairly certain that was not what (our child) had and we decided to look further.

We went to Children's Memorial in Chicago and . . . they diagnosed (our child) with 22Q13 Deletion (Phelan-McDermid Syndrome). . . .

In addition to our own knowledge and comfort, there have been specific benefits for (our child) receiving a diagnosis. When we were first looking for a diagnosis, (our child) was diagnosed with arachnoid cysts and neurologists had recommended yearly MRIs. Once we had the diagnosis we were instructed not to proceed with future MRIs as the diagnosis explained the brain phenomena. In addition, we were instructed to have a CT of (our child's) kidneys because problems are frequent in this population. Even learning simple, seemingly inconsequential, things proved helpful. We avoided the use of antifungal medication after learning that these kids just tend to have flaky toenails. . . .

In (our child's) case, we were able to avoid some costly and emotionally draining tests. I can also say that the diagnosis provided some peace of mind.

---

Etiology can be divided into two broad categories: genetic and acquired. Genetic causes are present at conception; acquired causes may be prenatal, perinatal, or postnatal in nature. In general, the closer in time an etiology is to conception, the more likely it is that it will affect more organ systems of the developing person and that those effects will produce a physically recognizable syndrome. Practically, this means that if an etiology has not yet been determined for an individual, a person who appears to have more body systems affected by the disorder is more likely to have an underlying genetic cause rather than an acquired cause.

## Common complications

Neurodevelopmental disorders tend to produce one or more of five general categories of common complications. These common complications include (1) intellectual disability; (2) neuromotor dysfunction; (3) seizure disorder; (4) psychiatric disorders; and (5) sensory impairment.

Though no estimates exist regarding the percentage of people with neurodevelopmental disorders having any of these particular complications,

**Table 5.1**  Complications of neurodevelopmental disorders associated with ID.

Neuromotor dysfunction: 20–30%
Seizure disorder: 15–30%
Behavioral disorders: 15–35%
Vision impairment: 17–25%
Hearing impairment: 20–32%

in the presence of ID, the likelihood of any one of the other four complications also being present is around 25% (Holder et al. 2007) (see Table 5.1).

As was discussed earlier, intellectual disability is characterized by significant limitations in adaptive functioning, an age of onset prior to 18, and is often associated with an IQ of less than 70.

Neuromotor dysfunction is most easily recognized as cerebral palsy, though it can take many forms. In many cases, this complication is brought on by a hypoxic injury to the fetal brain. Despite the fact that severe neuromotor dysfunction can significantly impair physical movement, coordination, and communication ability, many individuals who exhibit neuromotor dysfunction may not have ID and may be of average, above average, or even genius-level intelligence.

Seizure disorders of any type may manifest in patients with neurodevelopmental disorders. Though it is beyond the scope of this chapter to discuss the various types of seizure disorders in detail, dentists should familiarize themselves with various anti-seizure treatment modalities and their common side effects. Gingival hyperplasia, gastroesophageal reflux, bruxism, and osteoporosis are common medication side effects that may directly impact the oral health of the patient.

Psychiatric disorders commonly occur in this population, often manifesting as self-injurious behavior or aggressive behavior. Often these behaviors arise due to the patient's inability to adequately communicate with those around. Because the patient has a less precise repertoire of communication techniques, feelings of distress, discomfort, dislike, or displeasure may be acted out instead of verbally communicated. When confronted with aggressive or self-injurious behavior, it is important to determine whether these behaviors are a persistent characteristic of the patient or whether the behavior is relatively new. New behaviors tend to indicate a recently changed state such as new-onset pain and not an inherent personal trait.

It is not uncommon for patients with significant dental pain to exhibit these behaviors along with weight loss or weight gain due to dietary changes. Unfortunately, the psychiatric community may misinterpret these symptoms as a sign of depression, anxiety, or any number of other psychiatric disorders and may implement psychopharmacologic therapy inappropriately. Thus, the dental practitioner can play a significant role in redirecting inappropriate psychiatric care.

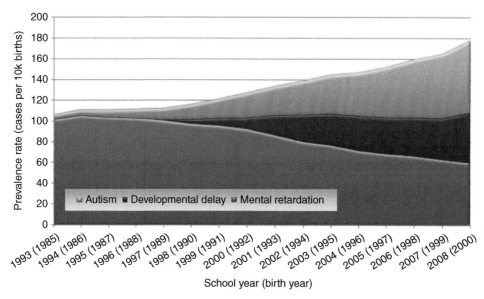

**Figure 5.2**  Prevalence rates for mental retardation, developmental delay, and autism for 8-year-olds for the years 1993–2008 (birth years 1985–2000), from U.S. Dept. of Education (IDEA) and CDC (birth) data.

Another very common psychiatric disorder associated with neurodevelopmental disorders is autism (or autism spectrum disorders). Though autism, much like intellectual disability, is often discussed as though it is a primary diagnosis, it is not. In the past decade, autism has gained much notoriety for its seemingly rapid increase in prevalence. While it appears as though some of this rise in the prevalence of autism may be attributed to a "relabeling" of individuals who in decades past may (correctly or incorrectly) have been given the diagnosis of mental retardation, it is certain that more children and adults are associated with autism spectrum disorders than at any other time in history (Shattuck 2006) (see Figure 5.2). As such, clinicians should familiarize themselves with autism spectrum disorders and be prepared to accommodate their practice for the behavioral and communication differences that are associated with these individuals.

Sensory impairments also tend to accompany many neurodevelopmental disorders. Sensory impairments tend to be limited to hearing and vision impairments, which occur independently in around 25% of people with ID. One myth that has been erroneous purveyed to some health care professionals is that there is a decrease in the ability to sense pain in these individuals. While the inability to feel pain has been described in the medical literature, it is an exceedingly rare phenomenon. As a rule, the perception of pain does not seem to be impaired in this patient population. What can be said to be different, in some cases, is the patient's reaction to

Box 5.2    Clinical vignette.

A 32-year-old male patient who had been receiving psychiatric treatment for worsening self-injurious behavior over the past 3 years presented to the dentist for a long-overdue comprehensive examination. Upon x-ray examination, eight dental abscesses were discovered.

Once treated, the patient's family immediately noticed a significant decrease in self-injurious behavior. Within 3 months, all episodes of self-injurious behavior had ceased and the patient was able to discontinue the anti-psychotic medications that had been prescribed by the treating psychiatrist.

pain, but pain is experienced nonetheless. Because the communication of pain may be different, clinicians should take extra precautions to ensure that their patients are not experiencing pain during dental procedures (see Box 5.2).

## Syndrome-specific conditions

As was stated previously, the closer the etiology of the disability occurs to time to conception, the more likely the etiology is to affect multiple organ systems. When various etiologies affect humans in similar patterns, they are classified as syndromes. The etiology of Down syndrome, for example is trisomy of the 21st chromosome. Its primary complications usually include ID. Additionally, sensory impairments are often present, along with mild neuromotor impairment. However, this only describes the complications due to the changes in the neurological system of people with Down syndrome. Many other organ systems in Down syndrome are also commonly affected. People with Down syndrome often have cardiac defects, thyroid issues, immunologic changes, and macroglossia occurring in conjunction with microstomia. Though not present in all people with Down syndrome, these syndrome-specific conditions occur in high enough frequencies that they should be investigated by the clinician, as they may be associated with secondary health consequences.

For the average clinician, the most significant type of syndrome-specific condition to consider is the cardiac defect (Table 5.2). In the United States, the three most common neurodevelopmental disorders are Down syndrome, fragile X syndrome, and fetal alcohol syndrome. Table 5.2 shows the extraordinary rates associated with these and two other relatively common neurodevelopemental disorders (Holder 2007). In fact, there are scores of known neurodevelopmental disorders that are associated with

**Table 5.2** Cardiac defect rates in common neurodevelopmental disorders.

Down syndrome: 40–50%
Fetal alcohol syndrome: 29–41%
Fragile X: up to 52%
Turner syndrome: up to 50%
Williams syndrome: up to 75%

cardiac defects. The specter of cardiac defects is so prevalent in this population that despite the recent changes in the American Heart Association guidelines regarding premedication, many dentists who treat people with developmental disorders opt to premedicate all of their patients with neurodevelopmental disorders until they have been examined and cleared by a cardiologist.

Other commonly occurring classes of syndrome-specific conditions that can affect dental care are malformations of the oropharynx and gastrointestinal tract, and abnormal collagen or bone composition. As with all of the common complications of neurodevelopmental disorders, the significance of many syndrome-specific conditions lies not necessarily with the condition itself but with the secondary health consequences that can arise because of them.

## Secondary health consequences

Secondary health consequences play a significant role in the on-going health of a person with a neurodevelopmental disorder. Secondary health consequences arise as a direct result of a complication or syndrome-specific condition associated with a particular disorder. For example, if a person with cerebral palsy who uses a wheelchair develops a decubitus ulcer, the ulcer is a secondary health consequence of the neuromotor dysfunction experienced by the patient. Secondary health consequences can build upon each other. For example, the decubitus ulcer could become infected and the infection could become systemic; each of these would be an additional secondary health consequence.

Unfortunately, people with developmental disorders often face multiple secondary health consequences as a result of their primary neurodevelopmental complications. These can significantly affect, or be affected by, disease processes in the oral cavity.

Intellectual disability, for example, can hinder a patient's ability to follow oral hygiene instructions or may impede the proper self-determination as to when it is beneficial to visit the dentist. Neuromotor dysfunction can hinder a person's ability to brush his or her own teeth, resulting in very poor oral hygiene. In many patients with cerebral palsy, spasticity can cause severe and persistent bruxism resulting in extraordinary loss of tooth structure. Seizure disorders can result in traumatic tooth avulsion, though perhaps more importantly, some medications used to treat seizures can result in gingival hyperplasia. Sensory impairments may interfere with a patient's understanding of hygiene instructions or treatment options. Behavioral conditions may interfere with a clinician's or direct support professional's willingness to treat the patient. Syndrome-specific conditions such as the microstomia, macroglossia, collagen defects, and immunological deficits associated with Down syndrome can create oral environments where periodontal disease will thrive. In people with Down syndrome, for example, periodontal disease is present in around 90% of patients (Pilcher 1998).

All of the above are examples of secondary health consequences that arise because of the primary complications associated with neurodevelopmental disorders. For a variety of social and physical factors, these secondary health consequences tend to develop faster and to a greater extent in patients with developmental disorders than in the general population. While clinicians will be called upon to treat these secondary health consequences, if it is possible to trace the genesis of the secondary health consequence to its primary cause, the primary factors may be addressed and, in doing so, future secondary consequences may be averted.

# INTELLECTUAL DISABILITY AND UNMET HEALTH NEEDS

Because intellectual disability is one of the most defining and prevalent characteristics of this patient population, it has been studied fairly extensively. Across all disciplines, ID tends to be correlated with poor health outcomes and a higher level of unmet health needs. Special Olympics has compiled data on thousands of athletes with intellectual disabilities in order to illustrate some of the unmet needs faced by these individuals (Table 5.3). Some of these data are noted in Table 5.3 (Corbin 2005).

**Table 5.3**  Unmet health needs vital statistics.

Vision: 25% myopic, 10% are presbyopic
Hearing: 30% fail hearing tests
Podiatry: 11% have athlete's foot, more than 50% wear the wrong size shoe
Bone health: 20% have low bone density
Metabolism: 53% are overweight or obese
Fitness: 22% need physical therapy
Medicine: 25% are taking medications that can have adverse side effects
Dentistry: 35% have untreated decay, 12% are in pain

# THE ORAL-SYSTEMIC CONNECTION

Though much has been written about the effect that oral health has on the rest of the body, there is perhaps no population where this aspect of oral health is more important than in people with developmental disorders. In general, dental care is consistently named as one of the most unmet health needs of this population. Consequently, the degree of oral pathology and thus the systemic effects of that pathology found in this population can be impressive. The examples below discuss many of the ways in which dental disease may impact other body systems or vice versa.

## Gastroesophageal reflux disease

Syndrome-specific conditions associated with neurodevelopmental disorders may include disorders of the gastrointestinal system. These conditions along with the medications frequently prescribed for this population may increase the likelihood that a patient with a developmental disorder will have gastroesophageal reflux disease (GERD). While many dentists might assume that GERD will be detected by a physician, in many cases, especially in nonverbal patients, a dentist may be the first to discover the telltale signs of GERD. Posterior enamel erosion such as that in Figure 5.3 is often a clear indication of GERD. In

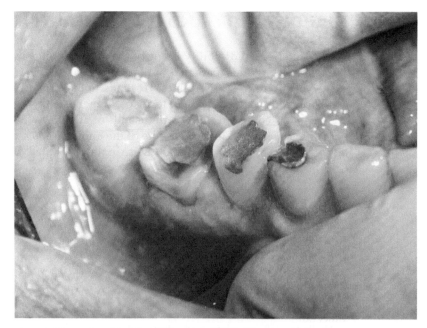

**Figure 5.3**  Posterior enamel erosion in a patient with a developmental disorder and GERD. Courtesy of the Underwood and Lee Clinic.

treating this patient population, it is of utmost importance to consider that if acid from the stomach has had this much of an effect on the teeth, it has likely had a significant effect on other structures of the esophagus and oropharynx. In this case, a gastrointestinal physician should be contacted with the recommendation of a follow-up endoscopy of the patient. As a result of this referral, secondary health consequences of GERD, such as esophagitis and esophageal neoplasm, can be prevented or treated early.

## Medications

According to some estimates, the average adult with ID can be on seven or more different medications (Holder et al. 2007). Very often these medications are used chronically and can produce significant side effects. Unfortunately, in many instances the medications have been prescribed or continued for inappropriate reasons. Because of the potential for adverse medication side effects in this population, the patient's medication regimen should be reexamined periodically by those treating the patient. Dentists can play a significant role in mitigating these effects, though this requires some investigation on the part of the dentist and a willingness to work in an interdisciplinary fashion with his or her physician counterparts.

There are hundreds of medications that can lead to xerostomia, stomatitis, caries, GERD, or gingival hyperplasia. If any of these symptoms are encountered in a patient with a developmental disorder, a quick review of the patient's medication regimen may reveal a medication that is contributing to the situation. If this is the case, the patient's physician should be notified of these effects, along with a recommendation that alternative treatment options be considered.

## Pain and behavior

In patients with intellectual disability, especially those who are nonverbal or have limited communication ability, the cause of new-onset behavior change is often related to undiagnosed pain or discomfort. Unfortunately most physicians and psychiatrists who are not familiar with this patient population (which is the majority of physicians and psychiatrists) are not aware of this. Therefore, the treating physician may look no further than treating the patient's behavior with psychoactive medications rather than performing an extensive workup for undiagnosed pain.

A dentist treating this population will often encounter patients who are in active pain or discomfort. Data from Special Olympics suggests that approximately 1 out of 8 athletes with ID is in active dental pain at any given time. Some data suggest that in a more significantly disabled population, potentially pain-causing lesions may be found in up to one-third of patients with neurodevelopmental disorders (Farman et al. 2003). Identifying and removing the cause of potential dental pain or gastrointestinal pain via collaboration with a gastrointestinal physician may have a significant effect upon the behavior of a patient with a developmental disorder. Thus, any time this occurs in a patient who is taking psychoactive medications, especially if the medication has been prescribed for a recent change in behavior, the dentist should contact the patient's primary care physician or psychiatrist and request another evaluation of the patient's behavior status. Anecdotal evidence suggests that removing causes of pain will reduce the need for behavioral control via medication.

## Osteoporosis

Because of syndrome-specific changes in bone metabolism or because of any number of medications (anti-seizure medications being a common culprit), patients with developmental disorders are at significant risk for the early development of osteoporosis. According to Special Olympics data, approximately 1 in 5 athletes with ID, at an average age of 24, will have abnormally low bone density. Some evidence suggests that dentists may be able to detect signs of osteoporosis on x-ray examination (Roberts et al. 2010). While these techniques are just coming to the fore, a dentist with this capability may be able to save a patient from a later long-bone fracture by working with the patient's physician to address the ostoeoporosis.

# GENERAL ANESTHESIA AND BEHAVIOR GUIDANCE/ MANAGEMENT

Behavior guidance and body movement management can often be one of the most challenging aspects of working with patients with developmental disorders. In one study, it was determined that over two-thirds of dentists who exclusively treat this population were failing to perform adequate x-ray examination and periodontal charting on their patients. The most cited reason for this lack of the most basic standard of care was the uncontrollable body movements of the patients (Farman et al. 2001). It is no wonder then that a dentist unfamiliar with body movement guidance and management techniques may move quickly to the employment of general anesthesia for no other purpose than behavior management. The result of this, however, is that approximately 25% of patients with ID who are served in the community are given general anesthesia for even the most routine of dental services (Dwyer 1998).

General anesthesia is an extraordinarily expensive means of behavior control. It also comes with morbidity and mortality risks that are not associated with other means of behavior control. Because of this, general anesthesia should be the last option with regard to behavior management. With proper utilization of behavior management techniques (Table 5.4), the

**Table 5.4**  Hierarchy of behavior guidance and management.

1.  In-office desensitization
2.  Gentle movement redirection
3.  Gentle hand-holding or head positioning
4.  Use of weighted blanket
5.  Limited use of wrist and/or ankle restraints
6.  Limited used of papoose restraint
7.  Oral sedation (of limited use)
8.  IV sedation
9.  General anesthesia

rate of use of general anesthesia can be decreased from 25% to less than 5% (Hood 2009).

There is a temptation among caregivers to interpret patient movement in the dental chair as dental phobia or a form of anxiety. This then leads to pressure on dentists to prescribe anxiolytics or other means of oral sedation in an effort to control patient behaviors. Unfortunately, in this patient population anxiolytics often have the paradoxical effect of disinhibiting the patient and accentuating his or her behaviors. This may move the clinician even closer to deciding to use general anesthesia. Thus, the prescribed use of anxioloytics should be carefully considered.

It is important for every dentist treating patients with developmental disorders to be able to differentiate between patient agitation and patient anxiety. While both may result in excessive patient movement, they are two very different behavioral mechanisms. Agitation occurs as a direct result of the sensations felt by the patient while receiving dental treatment. The resulting self-protective movement is almost reflexive. It is not a product of days or hours of phobic anticipation of dental treatment, as in the case of anxiety. In the case of the former, which is more often the case in this patient population, anxiolytics are not appropriate treatment and will likely only exacerbate patient behaviors. Ultimately, the use of both oral sedation and general anesthesia can have a place in the care of people with developmental disorders. It is, however, important for the clinician to safeguard against their inappropriate use.

## Interdisciplinary communication

If general anesthesia is used appropriately, it may provide an opportunity for the dentist to lead the health care team in providing comprehensive whole-person care. If the dentist has been unable to control behaviors to such an extent that general anesthesia is warranted, the odds are high that other clinicians have also been unable to render basic care to these individuals. In these cases it is unlikely that the patient has had a recent EKG, adequate breast or gynecological examination if female, prostate examination if male, endoscopy, or colonoscopy. If the dentist is going to order general anesthesia in order to provide dental care, it is in the best interest of the patient for the dentist to speak with the patient's primary care physician in order to coordinate any other services that the patient may not have been able to receive.

This coordination of services speaks to a larger issue with regard to caring for people with developmental disorders, the issue of interdisciplinary communication. Patients with developmental disorders are often unable to advocate effectively for themselves within the context of the health care system. Because of this, communication between the various health care professionals in that person's life is essential. Dentists can play a vital role in improving the quality of life for the patient, far beyond the borders of the oral cavity. The following are just a few examples of other professionals that dentists who treat patients with developmental disorders may contact and what some of the common issues are that they would discuss:

- Cardiology
  - Ruling out cardiac defect. Premedicating certain patients.
  - Treating hypertension detected prior to the dental visit.
- Gastroenterology
  - Recommending an upper endoscopy due to suspected GERD. Coordinating examinations with patients under general anesthesia.
  - Recommending changes to GERD medication regimen.
- Genetics
  - Establishing a neurodevelopmental diagnosis.
- Gynecology
  - Coordinating gynecological examination of patients under general anesthesia.
- Neurology
  - Recommending changes in anti-seizure medications because of gingival hyperplasia or suspected osteoporosis.
- Primary care
  - Coordinating care with any of the aforementioned specialists. Modifying anti-seizure, psychoactive, or other medications.
- Psychiatry
  - Recommending a reevaluation of psychoactive medications following the successful treatment of potentially pain-causing lesions.
- Speech therapy
  - Chewing and swallowing studies (reducing risk of aspiration) based on clinical suspicion during treatment.

## SUMMARY

This chapter discussed a number of themes that are pertinent to the overall health of people with developmental disorders. First, understanding the relationships between the various terms used to describe this population helps the clinician understand the basic characteristics of these patients so that he or she may have a more logical and consistent approach to patient care. Second, it is important to understand that this population has significant unmet health needs across many different disciplines. Third, it is also important to understand that proper dental care can affect a number of nondental systems of the body and that these effects should be considered when rendering care. Finally, interdisciplinary care is the key to better health care for people with developmental disorders, thus it is incumbent upon every dental professional to establish relationships with other health care professionals.

# REFERENCES

Corbin SB. (2005). *The Health and Healthcare of People with Intellectual Disabilities*. Washington, DC: Special Olympics.

Developmental Disabilities Assistance and Bill of Rights Act of 2000. (2000). Public Law 106-402, Subtitle A, Section 102(8)(a).

Dwyer RA. (1998). *Access to quality dental care for persons with developmental disabilities*. Chippewa Falls, WI: Northern Wisconsin Center for Developmentally Disabled.

Farman AB, Hood HD, Boggs KD, Cornett TS. (2001). The Hazelwood Study part I: Dental care of the institutionalized, profoundly cognitively impaired in the southeastern region of the United States. *Journal of the Southeastern Society of Pediatric Dentistry* 7(3):42–44.

Farman AB, Horsely B, Warr E, et al. (2003). Outcomes of digital x-ray mini-panel examinations for patients having mental retardation and developmental disability. *Dentomaxillofacial Radiology* 32(1):15–20.

Holder M. (2007). *Healthy Athletes MedFest: A Training Manual for Clinical Directors*. Washington, DC: Special Olympics.

Holder M, Hood H, Zelenski S, et al. (2007). *The Continuum of Quality Care Series*. Louisville, KY: American Academy of Developmental Medicine and Dentistry.

Hood HD. (2009). Underwood and Lee Clinic, unpublished clinical data.

Pilcher ES. (1998). Dental care for the patient with Down syndrome. *Down Syndrome Research and Practice* 5(2):111–116.

Rader R. (2007). The emergence of the American Academy of Developmental Medicine and Dentistry: Educating clinicians about the challenges and rewards of treating patients with special health care needs. *Pediatric Dentistry* 29(2):134–137.

Roberts MG, Graham J, Devlin H. (2010). Improving the detection of osteoporosis from dental radiographs using Active Appearance Models. *2010 IEEE International Symposium on Biomedical Imaging: From Nano to Macro*, 440–443.

Schalock RL, Borthwick-Duffy SA, Bradley VJ, et al. (2010). *Intellectual Disability: Definition, Classification, and Systems of Supports*, 11th ed. Washington, DC: American Association on Intellectual and Developmental Disabilities.

Schalock RL, Luckasson RA, Shogren KA, et al. (2007). The renaming of mental retardation: Understanding the change to the term intellectual disability. *Intellectual and Developmental Disabilities* 45(2):116–124.

Shattuck PT. (2006). The contribution of diagnostic substitution to the growing administrative prevalence of autism in U.S. special education. *Pediatrics* 117:1028–1037.

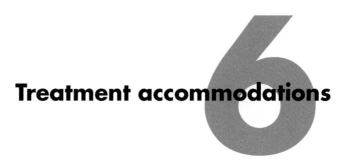

# Treatment accommodations

Debra Cinotti, DDS

## INTRODUCTION

Treatment accommodations for dental patients with developmental disorders (DDs) can be viewed as adaptations or modifications of customary practices to provide oral health care. The objective of incorporating accommodations is to provide quality treatment in a safe and effective manner, as well as providing a nonthreatening environment whenever feasible, thereby augmenting access to oral health care.

Patients with DDs experience access-to-care issues in part because the health care provider is intimidated by or lacks knowledge about meeting the treatment needs of persons with DD. One initiative set forth to increase the number of oral health care providers trained to provide treatment to persons with DD is a change in the educational standards for predoctoral dental students adopted by the Commission on Dental Accreditation (CODA). CODA "serves the public by establishing, maintaining and applying standards that ensure the quality and continuous improvement of dental and dental-related education and reflect the evolving practice of dentistry. The scope of the Commission on Dental Accreditation encompasses dental, advanced dental and allied dental education programs" (ADA 2010). CODA has modified its standards to mandate that the dental graduate "must be competent in assessing the treatment needs of patients with special needs" (ADA 2010).

*Treating the Dental Patient with a Developmental Disorder*, First Edition.
Edited by Karen A. Raposa and Steven P. Perlman.
© 2012 John Wiley & Sons, Inc. Published 2012 by John Wiley & Sons, Inc.

While these educational changes are commendable for future oral health care providers, the current provider workforce can also become skilled, knowledgeable, and comfortable in the delivery of quality care to persons with DDs. It is important to remember that the Americans with Disabilities Act (AwDA) requires "reasonable modifications in policies, practices, and procedures" enabling persons with disabilities equal opportunity to receive the goods and services available to others. Specifically, doctors' offices, classified as places of public accommodation, are covered by regulations set forth in Title 3 of the AwDA. Becoming familiar with Title 3 of the AwDA will assist health care providers to understand their obligation to provide health care to individuals with DD (U.S. Department of Justice 2011).

Becoming learned in the types of treatment accommodations considered for the DD patient facilitates the dental provider's ability to deliver safe and effective oral health care to these individuals. Earlier chapters discussed obtaining pertinent information (such as medical, dental, and social histories) prior to treatment as well as how to determine if treatment accommodations are necessary. This chapter will focus on what types of accommodations may be necessary for the DD patient, as learned from information obtained from the caregiver interview as well as patient experiences from previous dental/medical visits. Accommodations may be necessary to commence treatment as well as provide treatment. Take into consideration the intellectual capacity, behavioral challenges, mobility constraints, neuromuscular limitations, uncontrolled body movements, and medical profile of a patient that would benefit from adjustments to routine procedures (NIDCR 2011). For example, how does the dental provider obtain informed consent from a patient with DD? What accommodations should be taken to control stimuli in the dental office, such as noise? What accommodations are available for consideration to support the physically challenged patient's ability to receive care? Each of these circumstances will be discussed, providing the dental practitioner with useful means to enhance his or her knowledge of the delivery of care to the DD patient.

## ACQUISITION OF INFORMED CONSENT

Informed consent in health care refers to an agreement by the patient to receive specified procedures after receiving detailed information about the nature of the proposed procedures, other treatment options available, and the risks and benefits associated with these procedures (ADA 2010). As described in the *Miller-Keane Encyclopedia & Dictionary of Medicine, Nursing & Allied Health*, informed consent is based on the principles of autonomy and privacy and must satisfy seven different criteria: "(1) competence to understand and to decide, (2) voluntary decision making, (3) disclosure of material information, (4) recommendation of a plan, (5) comprehension of terms (3) and (4), (6) decision in favor of a plan, and (7) authorization of the plan" (*Miller-Keane* 2003). In addition, the individual providing consent must be of a certain age (ADA 2010). Informed consent is obtained before services are rendered. However, it is important to note that the laws and requirements governing informed consent are state driven and may be different for different types of procedures (Stein 2007).

When treating a DD patient, first determine the "decisional capacity" of that patient. Not all persons with DD lack ability to make informed decisions. Furthermore, an individual's ability to comprehend may vary with the complexity of the decision to be made. For example, a person may be able to comprehend and consent to an initial examination but not comprehend the risks and benefits of a proposed surgical intervention. Therefore, it is important to establish the patient's ability to fully understand the information provided. "The capacity to make health care decisions has been defined as the ability to understand the information about a proposed care plan, appreciate the consequences of a decision, and reach and communicate an informed decision" (Beltran 1996). As Beltran so aptly stated, "There is a need to balance protection from harm with the patient's right to self-determination. This balancing requires skilled listening, the proper level of advocacy from caregivers, and pragmatic models of shared decision making" (*Mosby's Medical Dictionary* 2009). A DD patient with full decisional capacity should provide informed consent for him- or herself. A DD patient with diminished capacity will either require assistance or depend completely on another person to provide informed consent. This other person should be the patient's guardian or surrogate decision maker (an identified individual or organization appointed to assist or make decisions regarding the welfare of the DD patient, when the patient does not have a guardian). Once again, laws determining guardianship of a person with developmental disabilities vary from state to state. State law may require that when an individual becomes of "legal" age, a court order is necessary to (1) determine diminished decision-making capacity and the need to appoint guardianship, and (2) grant approval for those seeking the role of guardian.

Once it is determined who will give informed consent, the dental provider should determine if the current policies and procedures routinely followed in the office are acceptable for the patient with limited decision-making capabilities. Often, implied informed consent is accepted for the initial examination visit. Implied informed consent is when a patient permits care without a formal agreement between the patient and health care provider. When a patient calls and schedules an appointment, it is implied that the patient has consented to the treatment visit (Ferguson et al. 1996). However, for the patient who is dependent on a guardian or surrogate to provide informed consent, it is recommended to obtain written informed consent for all forms of treatment, including general routine care, utilization of behavioral guidance aids, and surgical treatments.

Patients who reside in a facility and not with a guardian may be escorted for treatment with a caretaker who does not have authority to provide informed consent. To obtain informed consent for these individuals consider the following options:

1. If a patient's guardian lives within distance of the providing dental care facility, require the guardian to attend the visits requiring consent for treatment.
2. If a patient's guardian lives a far distance from the dental care facility (which is a common occurrence), obtain informed consent from the guardian/surrogate prior to the appointment. Informed consent should be obtained for the initial examination, diagnosis, and treatment planning visit, including informed consent for behavioral guidance aids. These consent forms should include specific information describing the nature of the treatment, alternative treatments available, and associated risks and benefits. After the initial examination and diagnosis visit, the proposed treatment plan would require informed consent as well. To help facilitate this process, another option for these individuals is to formulate a memorandum of understanding (MOU) between the residential facility, the patient's guardian, and the dental care provider (Ferguson 2005). The MOU may serve as a contract of informed consent allowing designated treatment to be rendered based on specific criteria described in the MOU. The MOU document would have to include all information required of informed consent.

With respect to consent for behavioral guidance aids, a separate informed consent form may be obtained. This form should describe the protocol utilized to determine if behavioral aids will be used, as well as a description of these aids and the associated risks and benefits with use. The form should also define the time period for which the consent is valid and the opportunities and procedures to withdraw the consent prior to the expiration date. An "extended" informed consent for utilization of behavioral guidance aids enables the dental care provider to perform treatment with these aids over multiple visits. This facilitates care especially for patients residing in a residential facility and not accompanied to the dental visits by a guardian or surrogate individual authorized to provide informed consent. It goes without saying that the standards for utilizing behavioral guidance must be followed.

In summary, informed consent is essential for any patient and may require special consideration for individuals with developmental disabilities. However, the process does not have to be a difficult one. If the DD patient has full decision-making capacity, follow standard procedure to obtain informed consent. If the DD patient has limited decision-making capacity, have the guardian present to assist the patient in giving informed consent. Obtain both signatures on the informed consent. If the patient has no decision-making capacity, identify the guardian/surrogate and obtain informed consent from that individual.

# ACCOMMODATIONS TO MANAGE
# GENERAL OFFICE STIMULI

Persons without intellectual disabilities may experience anxiety or other fearful reactions in anticipation of their dental visit. However, upon entering the office, most often these individuals understand the cause of their uneasy feelings and are able to control their reaction to office stimuli. Office stimuli can refer to a wide array of details that are commonplace to the dental office. Examples of stimuli include "the white coat" worn by the dental provider, high activity within the office, the sounds of the drill, the smells of medicaments, and the sight of dental instruments, just to name a few. However, the DD patient may not have the cognitive capacity to understand or control his or her reaction upon entering the dental office. Perceiving the dental environment negatively, these individuals may present with challenging behaviors, ranging from self-injurious behavior to aggressive outbursts and attempts to leave the office.

As a first step in managing impulsivity and negative reactions by the DD patient to the dental office, understanding the triggers for his or her behaviors would help to define what accommodations to make. This is one of the core principles in functional analysis of behaviors whose principles are beyond the scope of this chapter. Suffice it to say that functional analysis helps to determine the correlation between specific stimuli and responses to that stimuli. If the triggers are identified, the patient may be taught positive coping mechanisms and/or effective changes to the office environment can be made. A simple list of accommodations to consider for control of general office stimuli include:

- Minimize heightened activity, noise.
- Schedule appointments during the least busy time of day (perhaps the first or last appointment of the day) for patients who react to a busy office environment.
- Schedule short appointments.
- Avoid scheduling the DD patient with other highly active patients. For example, avoid scheduling with a pediatric patient who may be very vocal during care.
- Schedule the first appointment as an introduction appointment to the dental team and the physical space (operatory). This appointment should be kept short and positive. Do not render oral care during this appointment.
- When interacting with the patient directly, avoid rapid movements or rapid speech; rather, move and speak in a calm manner.
- Wear a protective coat of a different color for the patient who responds negatively to the traditional doctor's white coat.
- Identify comforting items that help the patient to relax; for example, perhaps listening to music or holding a comfort toy. Not only might this

distract the patient from anxiety-producing office noise and work but also includes an activity that is part of the patient's daily routine, providing familiarity and comfort.

# ACCOMMODATIONS FOR THE TREATMENT OPERATORY

The above is a partial list and sample of many such accommodations that might be considered for the anxious DD patient to control office stimuli. But what about the actual treatment session and associated armamentarium? Does the sight of the instruments create anxiety? Does the patient have a tendency to touch or grab new objects? Suggestions follow to meet the challenges presented by operatory stimuli and facilitate delivery of dental care.

## Setting up the operatory

The operatory should be fully prepared prior to the patient's arrival to prevent disruption during the treatment visit. This is desirable for any patient visit, but especially for patients who may have a limited attention span or ability to cooperate. The following should be present (Ferguson 2005):

- Instrument tray appropriate for the procedure.
- Appropriate-size toothbrush.
- Mouth props to assist with opening.
- 4 by 4 Gauze/cotton rolls.
- Patient mirror (for patient to observe procedure).
- Aids helpful in occupying patient's hands (toy, doll).
- Medical immobilization aids based on information received about behavior compliance.

Consider utilizing the toothbrush prior to any other instrumentation. A toothbrush is often the first "instrument" used at the DD patient's visit. This is especially helpful if the patient receives daily home care, as it is a familiar "tool." However, it is an unfortunate reality that many DD patients are lacking in daily home care. Nevertheless, the toothbrush can be used to introduce other instruments into "play." Let the patient watch you with a patient mirror. The patient mirror is a common element used in pediatric dentistry and acts to engage the patient in the visit and remove the mystery from what is occurring. Utilization of the patient mirror or any aid will be dependent on the patient's cognitive abilities and compliance behavior.

If you have information suggesting that "seeing" the instruments produces a negative response, cover the instruments with a bib or other covering to keep from the patient's sight upon entering the operatory. Maintain the instrument tray out of the patient's view for the duration of the procedure. Likewise, if the patient has a tendency to grab or touch new objects, keep the instruments out of the patient's view or, at the very least, out of the patient's reach.

In some instances, the dental light is bothersome to the patient. Determine if the patient becomes more relaxed with the room lights dimmed and use of a head lamp as opposed to the overhead dental light. For some patients, allowing them to wear sunglasses resolves this issue, while at the same time making the patients feel special.

Mouth props or mouth rests are used to help the patient maintain an open mouth. They come in variable shapes, sizes, and materials. Some may contain latex, others are latex free. Some are disposable, others reusable. Standard types used include the bite block and mouth gag or mouth molt. Other choices also exist that may seem less intrusive and therefore, less threatening and more comfortable for the patient to tolerate. One such choice is a wedge-shaped handle that is made of a dense foam with a wooden core (Specialized Care Co., Inc. 2011) (Figure 6.1). The operator places the wedge-shaped end over the occlussal surfaces of the teeth in the upper and lower arch, stabilizing it by holding the other end.

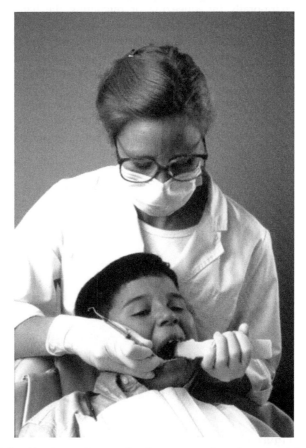

**Figure 6.1**   Mouth rest. Reprinted with permission from Specialized Care Co.

This option comes in two sizes based on the thickness of the foam—the thicker handle is used for patients having a strong or "heavy" bite. Another nonconventional choice may be a soft, thickset, rubber-like handle of a child's toothbrush, which can be used in similar fashion to the foam handle described above.

The bite-block type of rest is a triangulated block placed intra-orally (Figure 6.2). It is shaped to fit against the cheek mucosa, covering the occlussal surfaces of the upper and lower arch. Depending on the manufacturer, some have handles (tab or wraparound found at Specialized Care Company, Inc. 2011), while others have no handles (Hu-Friedy 2011).

The mouth gag or mouth molt is a scissor or ratchet-type appliance that rests outside the mouth on the patient's cheek with extended "wings" that are placed onto the dentition's occlussal surfaces of the upper and lower arch. As it is positioned outside the mouth, it may work best for patients with a strong gag reflex. In addition, the initial placement of this device does not require the patient to open wide. Just enough of an opening to properly place the "wings" is required. Once placed, the device is opened extra-orally by squeezing or ratcheting the handles together. (Refer to Chapter 10 for a picture of this device in use.)

In conclusion, when choosing a mouth rest, a number of variables should be considered, including the patient's tolerance level for an intra-oral versus an extra-oral device, the ease with which the device can be placed, the patient's gag reflex, strength of the patient's bite reflex, and the anxiety level of the patient—is one device better received than another? Whichever device is chosen, the dental provider must learn how to place the device as well as the risks and benefits of each one.

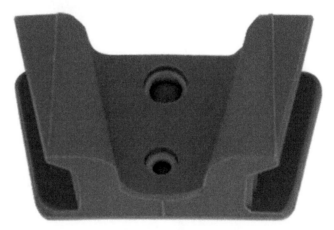

**Figure 6.2**  Mouth props. Reprinted with permission from Specialized Care Co.

## Creating a secure environment

Establishing a familiar environment and providing comfort aids helps to create a secure, nonthreatening milieu that may reduce the patient's anxiety and ability to accept treatment. Accommodations that encourage familiarity include:

- Maintaining continuity of care using the same dental team members at each appointment. This gives an opportunity for the patient to develop a trust between him- or herself and the dental provider and assistant.
- Allowing the caregiver/parent into the treatment room. However, establish guidelines for the role of the accompanying person prior to the dental visit to avoid disruption of the treatment session. Allow the caregiver to hold the patient's hands during treatment if this produces a calm demeanor for the patient. Often, the caregiver/guardian can provide reassurance to the patient with soothing words of encouragement. As the patient already trusts this individual, this trust may be transferred to the treatment team by association. Talking to the patient, however, should be limited to the treating provider while the patient is in the operatory. This will limit the potential for unintentional but inappropriate statements that may inadvertently frighten or distract the patient.
- Utilizing the same treatment room, preferably one furthest away from the "busyness" of the office. Consistency supports the development of trust between the patient and his or her environment.

Providing comfort aids can also help to lessen a negative response to the operatory setting. Learn what types of aids encourage cooperation in the home, school, or other social settings. Aids that are associated with enjoyment, calm, or other positive emotional responses can prove to be very effective in a dental treatment visit. Comfort aids can include holding onto a special toy; listening to music with earphones; lying with a pillow either as support to feel safer in the chair or to rest the head; or holding a known, familiar object when lying down.

Another aid that has been shown to help DD patients adapt positively to new environments is Snoezelen MSE (multi-sensory environments). DD individuals often lack the ability to regulate their response to sensory input or stimuli. Those of us who have control over our responses choose daily what stimuli we will react to and what stimuli we will ignore, as well as how we will respond. This is done without much thought to the neurological input necessary to achieve this control. Snoezelen MSE provides an opportunity for persons with DD to have more control over their responses, enhance communication skills, and, therefore, participate in settings otherwise perceived as threatening (Snoezelen Multi-Sensory Environments 2011).

Snoezelen MSE consists of specialized sensory equipment and materials that provide the DD individual with an array of primary sensory stimulation, including a "blend of sights, sounds, textures, aromas and motion" that the patient can control (Snoezelen Multi-Sensory Environments 2011). It can be used as a relaxation and transitioning tool to help DD individuals adapt to the stimuli of a dental office. An example of a Snoezelen product is a bubble tube that provides visual and tactile stimulation. Bubbles move up and down a water tube. Gazing at this movement is also thought to promote relaxation. Another Snoezelen product is a fiber optic light spray. There are different spray sets to choose from, each thought to affect mood elevation and/or relaxation. To learn more about Snoezelen products you can visit their Web site at http://www.snoezeleninfo.com/fiberOptics.asp.

Fidget toys are another aid used to reduce stress and enhance the ability to focus. Fidget toys are often used in therapies for children with attention deficit/hyperactivity disorder and autism. The toys come in all shapes and sizes. For the dental environment, fidget toys can be used to occupy the patient's hands as well as a distraction from other negatively perceived stimuli. This in turn calms the DD patient and actually may enhance his or her ability to focus. Fidget toys can be viewed on the web simply by searching "fidget toys."

# PROTECTIVE STABILIZATION AS A COPING MECHANISM

The term "protective stabilization" is considered to be a form of behavioral guidance and generally refers to "the restriction of patient's freedom of movement, with or without the patient's permission, to decrease risk of injury while allowing safe completion of treatment" (American Academy of Pediatric Dentistry 2011). Behavior guidance principles, along with the risks and benefits of protective stabilization techniques, are covered in detail in an earlier chapter. However, when thinking about treatment accommodations and utilization of protective stabilization to provide treatment in a safe and effective manner, one should also recognize that some of these techniques may actually calm or relax the patient. Examples might include the placement of a pillow strategically between the patient and the arm of the dental chair, restricting patient movement on the dental chair, providing a secure feeling for the patient; utilization of a pedi-wrap as a "blanket," the perception of "blanket" being a positive, comforting, and familiar one; or the use of arm stabilizers, assisting with uncontrollable spasticity, helping the patient to feel in control. In conclusion, do not discount protective stabilization as a means to relax the patient. For some DD individuals, relaxation achieved by protective stabilization may be perceived as less intimidating than sedation or general anesthesia. However, it is important to understand the indications, contraindications, and precautions necessary when using protective stabilization. It is essential to evaluate the patient's response to any technique used. Any decision made to utilize behavior guidance techniques should be based on a benefit versus risk evaluation (American Academy of Pediatric Dentistry 2011), and informed consent must be obtained from the appropriate individual(s).

## ACCOMMODATIONS FOR THE PHYSICALLY CHALLENGED

Some individuals with DD will present with physical disabilities that may require accommodation to customary practices. Such individuals might be those with cerebral palsy, muscular dystrophy, scoliosis, or paralysis. Others may have sensory deprivation. Specific disabilities may present with specific physical challenges that are best managed with specific treatment techniques to facilitate safe and effective care. The provider can become familiar with these needs through the information gathered prior to initiating treatment. Nevertheless, there are general accommodations to take into consideration that include, but are not limited to, the following:

- Maintain a clear pathway for wheelchairs and for the patient who may have an unsteady gait but remains ambulatory.
- Position pillows or pads to support the patient's body in the dental chair.
- Place the patient in a nonstressful posture, being careful not to force retracted limbs in an extended position.
- Utilize appropriate protective stabilization devices to provide a safe and secure environment.
- For those patients with sensory deprivations, such as visual or hearing loss, adopt communication techniques utilized by the patient's care-giver(s). This may involve utilization of tactile sensation for the visually impaired or adjustment of hearing aids or lip reading for those with diminished hearing.
- Be prepared to assist the patient in and out of the dental chair.
- Be mindful that not all physically challenged individuals have intellectual disabilities.

## CONCLUSION

Individuals with developmental disabilities are as varied in their present-ing needs as those without. It is important to recognize that not all persons with a developmental disorder have an intellectual disability. Some indi-viduals with DD require no change in customary practice routine, while others require some assistance, and still others depend on a third party for all decisions and care.

In general, however, persons with DD are faced with access-to-care issues in part because the health care provider is intimidated by or lacks knowledge about meeting the treatment needs of persons with DD. However, as presented above, dental practitioners can become learned in the types of treatment accommodations considered for the DD patient and deliver safe and effective oral health care to these individuals.

# REFERENCES

American Academy of Pediatric Dentistry Clinical Affairs Committee—Behavior Management Subcommittee; American Academy of Pediatric Dentistry Council on Clinical Affairs. (2011). Guideline on behavior guidance for the pediatric dental patient. Reference Manual 33(6 11/12):161–173.

American Dental Association (ADA) Council on Dental Practice, Division of Legal Affairs. (2010). Dental Records. Available at http://www.ada.org/sections/professionalResources/pdfs/dentalpractice_dental_records.pdf Accessed October 1, 2011.

Beltran JE. (1996). "Shared decision making: The ethics of caring and best respect" Bioethics Forum, 12:17–25.

Commission on Dental Education, Accreditation Standards for Dental Education Programs, Clinical Sciences Standard. (2010). American Dental Association. Accessed September 25, 2011, from http://www.ada.org/sections/educationAndCareers/pdfs/predoc.pdf, pp. 2–24.

Commission on Dental Education, Accreditation Standards for Dental Education Programs. (2010). American Dental Association. Accessed September 25, 2011, from http://www.ada.org/sections/educationAnd Careers/pdfs/predoc.pdf (Mission Statement, p. 2).

Ferguson F. (2005). Standards of Care for Patients with Special Needs.

Ferguson F, Cinotti DA, Kim W, Berentsen BJ. (1996). Facilitation of informed consent for agency residents with developmental disabilities. *Journal of Special Care Issues in Dentistry* 16(1):15–17.

Hu-Friedy Mouth Props and Gags. (2011). Accessed October 13, 2011, from http://www.hu-friedy.com/product/itemGroup.aspx?groupID=MPG&cat egoryID=Surgical.

*Miller-Keane Encyclopedia & Dictionary of Medicine, Nursing & Allied Health*, 7th ed. (2003). Informed consent. Accessed October 1, 2011, from http://medical-dictionary.thefreedictionary.com/informed+consent.

*Mosby's Medical Dictionary*, 8th ed. (2009). Informed consent. Accessed October 1, 2011, from http://medical-dictionary.thefreedictionary.com/informed+consent.

National Institute of Dental and Craniofacial Research, National institutes of Health. (2011). Continuing education: Practical oral care for people with developmental disabilities. Accessed October 8, 2011, from http://

www.nidcr.nih.gov/OralHealth/Topics/DevelopmentalDisabilities/ ContinuingEducation.htm.

Snoezelen multi-sensory environments. (2011). Accessed October 13,2011, from http://www.snoezeleninfo.com/whatIsSnoezelen.asp.

Specialized Care Co., Inc. Mouth Props and Mouth Rests (2011). Accessed October 13, 2011, from http://www.specializedcare.com/shop/pc/viewcategories.asp? idcategory=18.

Stein GL. (2007). Advance directives and advance care planning for people with intellectual and physical disabilities. Accessed October 1, 2011, from http:// aspe.hhs.gov/daltcp/reports/2007/adacp.htm.

U.S. Department of Justice. (2011). Civil Rights Division, Disability Rights Section, Americans with Disabilities Act. Accessed September 25, 2011, from http://www.ada.gov/t3hilght.htm.

# 7

# The exam/hygiene appointment

## Ann-Marie C. DePalma, CDA, RDH, MEd, FADIA, FAADH and Karen A. Raposa, RDH, MBA

All patients who present to the dental practice have unique histories, challenges, and preferences. Patients with developmental disorders are no different and need to be treated with open minds and hearts. Treating these patients will provide dental teams with unlimited rewards. This chapter will discuss:

- Strategies to prepare for a successful exam/hygiene appointment.
- Techniques for developing a team approach.
- Approaches for guiding the patient through the hygiene appointment.
- Suggestions for follow-ups and championing opportunities.

Treating the patient with a developmental disorder begins with the initial contact by the parent or caregiver. Depending on the practice, this contact may occur via telephone or internet registration. If the initial patient contact occurs through the internet, a phone call from the practice to the parent/caregiver should be initiated as soon as possible. As part of a "best practice" protocol, when a patient contacts a dental office for a new patient appointment, care must be taken to ensure that the patient is treated with respect and thoughtfulness (DePalma & Raposa 2010). All team members who have this initial contact need to be well informed regarding the dental practice's philosophy and treatment protocols. Team meetings, huddles, and continuing education programs that focus on new patient appointments are vital to the practice and can help enhance communication skills among

*Treating the Dental Patient with a Developmental Disorder*, First Edition.
Edited by Karen A. Raposa and Steven P. Perlman.
© 2012 John Wiley & Sons, Inc. Published 2012 by John Wiley & Sons, Inc.

the doctor, team members, and patient. These activities are especially important when working with patients with developmental disorders.

During this initial phone contact, the dental professional should explain that a welcome packet will be sent to the caregiver's attention. This packet should contain:

- A welcome letter explaining the practice philosophy.
- A review of the patient contact information obtained during the phone interview.
- Home care tips and skills to practice for the first visit.
- Patient information and interview forms.
- Office brochure and/or social story.

A social story can be produced by taking photos of all areas of the office and team, including the front of the office, the waiting area, and so forth, and putting them into a PowerPoint, Word or Adobe file. This will allow the addition of the name of each dental professional and room in the practice. The story can also be personalized by adding the patient's name to the story. This will help the patient to feel as if he or she already "knows" the practice before actually arriving.

In addition to traditional medical and dental history forms, a patient interview form (Figure 7.1) should be completed and returned to the office so that a telephone interview appointment can be scheduled to review the form. This separate patient information form will describe in more detail the patient's abilities relative to his or her disorder. It may include, but is not limited to, information such as:

- Type of disorder/diagnosis along with associated medical issues including seizure activity.
- Previous dental experiences.
- Daily oral care regimens, including times and locations.
- Oral habits, including those involving nonedible objects.
- Parent/caregiver's goals for dental treatment—present and future.
- Allergies, food sensitivities and/or aversions.
- Bladder or bowel adaptations.
- Physical function.
- Level of communication.
- Sensory abilities of sight and sound.
- Psychological status.
- Reward therapies used.
- Sensory stimulations.

Once this information is completed and received by the dental practice, a telephone interview can be scheduled to review the information provided. The phone call itself should take place during a scheduled appointment time when the practice representative can discuss the patient's abilities, questions, and concerns in detail. The time devoted to obtaining this information helps show the patient and parent/caregiver that the

DR. PHILIP M. ROBITAILLE

PATIENT INFORMATION (please print)

_____

Date: _____

## PERSONAL INFORMATION:

Name: _____

Address: _____

City: _____ State: _____ Zip Code: _____

Phone: (home) _____ (work) _____

Email Address: _____

Date of Birth:_____ / _____ /_____ Age: _____ Height: _____ Weight: _____

## PERSON TO CONTACT IN CASE OF EMERGENCY:

Name:_____ Relationship:_____

Address (if different from above): _____

_____

Phone: (home) _____ (work) _____

Current physician: _____

Phone: _____

## MEDICAL INFORMATION:

Describe the nature of your disability:

_____

_____

Are you currently taking any MEDICATIONS? YES/NO

If YES, what medications: _____

_____

Describe side effects of current medications: _____

_____

Have you ever had SEIZURES? YES/NO

If YES, date of last seizure: _____

Describe the type of seizure: _____

**Figure 7.1**   Supplemental form for patients with developmental disorders.

Do you have any ALLERGIES? YES/NO

If YES, please list: _____

_____

Do you have any FOOD SENSITIVITIES OR AVERSIONS? YES/NO

If YES, please list: _____

_____

Do you have any BLADDER or BOWEL ADAPTATIONS? YES/NO

Please list any adaptations: _____

_____

Are there any precautions we should be aware of regarding bladder/bowel control? _____

_____


## DENTAL EXPERIENCE:

Have you had any dental experiences? YES/NO

If YES, please describe: _____

_____

Do you have a dental experience at home on a daily basis? YES/NO

If YES, please describe: _____

_____

How would you describe your tolerance for dental experiences? Good/Fair/Poor

Do you use a powered toothbrush or a manual toothbrush? YES/NO

What are your dental health goals? _____

_____


## ORAL HABITS:

How often are you snacking during the day? _____

Is food used as a reward during therapy? _____

If YES, what types of food do you prefer? _____

Do you need to chew for sensory stimulation? YES/NO

If YES, how often per day? _____

If YES, what materials do you chew on? _____

Do you have a tendency to put nonedible items in your mouth? YES/NO

If YES, please describe: _____

**Figure 7.1** (Cont'd).

## PHYSICAL FUNCTIONING:

Are you currently working or attending school? _____

If YES, how long is your average work or school day? _____

Do you have difficulty breathing? _____

Do you have normal range of motion in the following?
Right arm: YES/NO
Left arm: YES/NO
If NO. please describe: _____

_____

Describe your strength (circle all that apply):
Upper body: Weak/Average/Strong
Left side: Weak/Average/Strong
Right side: Weak/Average/Strong

## SENSATION:

Is any part of your body paralyzed? YES/NO
Can you feel hot and cold normally? YES/NO

If YES to any of the above, please explain: _____

_____

## COMMUNICATION:

Receptive communication level: High/Medium/Low
Expressive communication level: High/Medium/Low
Can patient make needs known to dental team? YES/NO
Do you have difficulty speaking or communicating? YES/NO
Do others have difficulty understanding you? YES/NO
Do you have difficulty remembering things? YES/NO
Do you have difficulty in learning new things? YES/NO
Do you have difficulty following directions? YES/NO
Do you have difficulty hearing? YES/NO

If you answered YES to any of these questions, please explain: _____

_____

_____

Useful phrases or words that work best with patient? _____

_____

Does patient use nonverbal communication? YES/NO
If YES: Mayer Johnson Symbols/Sign Language/Picture Exchange Communication System (PECS)/ Sentence Board or Gestures

**Figure 7.1** (*Cont'd*).

Will you be bringing a communication system with you? YES/NO

Are there any symbols/signs that we can have available to assist with communication? _____

_____

## VISION:

Do you wear glasses? YES/NO
Do you wear contacts? YES/NO

Please mark any of the following that are true about your vision:
Double vision: YES/NO

Visual perceptual problems: YES/NO
Can only see to one side: YES/NO
If YES, which side? Left/Right

## HEARING:

Do you have a hearing impairment? YES/NO
Do you wear a hearing aid? YES/NO
If YES, please explain: _____

_____

## BEHAVIOR/EMOTIONS:

Impulsive? YES/NO
Do you become easily frustrated? YES/NO
Do you become angry easily? YES/NO
Do you ever physically/verbally lose control? YES/NO

Please give details to any question that you answered YES to: _____
_____
_____

What are the best ways to help you gain control? _____
_____

Behavior to be discouraged: _____
_____

PLEASE GIVE ANY ADDITIONAL INFORMATION THAT MAY HELP US TO PREPARE FOR A SUCCESSFUL DENTAL EXPERIENCE: _____
_____
_____
_____
_____
_____
_____

**Figure 7.1** (Cont'd).

practice is genuinely interested in understanding the patient's needs and has a desire to establish a positive and trusting relationship. Upon completion of the interview, the first visit with the office can be scheduled. The parent/caregiver should be asked what time of day is appropriate for the appointment, if any coping or comforting devices are needed by the patient in new situations, and if another adult can accompany the patient and parent/caregiver for additional behavioral supports during the appointment.

At the initial visit, the dental professional should discuss a goal for that visit with both the patient and parent/caregiver. The goal should be very simple (i.e., getting the patient to sit in the dental chair and allow the practitioner to look in the mouth without any instruments). Once this is accomplished, more and more difficult tasks can be added. Patients with developmental disorders are often distressed when less familiar practitioners are added to their treatments; therefore, it is best to keep clinical team treating the patient to a minimum and as constant as possible. As the patient begins to trust the dental professional team, additional team members can be added to the patient's care in the event the original clinician is not available. In understanding a patient's individual needs, the dental professional can be successful by tailoring treatment to suit the patient's abilities rather than disabilities (DePalma & Raposa 2010).

Prior to the first appointment and at each subsequent appointment, the patient should be introduced to home care tips and procedures that can be practiced at home in order to prepare for the next visit (e.g., practice placing a radiographic film or dental mirror in the mouth). The patient should never leave the office without a skill to be practiced for the next visit. This first appointment should be a trust-building appointment. Its primary purpose is to establish trust with the patient and parent/caregiver. This allows the patient and others involved in the patient's care to know that the practice is genuinely concerned about them. It should include a review of the medical, dental, and social information, provide orientation to the practice and dental team, and include a brief exam. The patient and/or parent/caregiver should be asked where the oral examination should occur—many developmentally challenged patients feel apprehensive in the dental chair. The location of this brief exam can be in the reception area, consultation office, operatory, team lounge, or anywhere the patient is most comfortable. Remember there is no "rule" that says an exam has to take place in the dental operatory; it could even be performed in the car if that is the only place the patient will allow the examination. The goal for the next appointment would be to allow the examination to take place in the dental office.

The dental professional should follow the "tell-show-do" protocol; not asking the patient if it is okay to proceed but telling what will happen, showing the patient what will happen, and then proceeding to do the event. A key to building a trusting relationship during the initial appointment involves a reward system. During the phone interview, the appropriate reward system for the patient should be gleaned from the parent/caregiver and should be included in the materials that are needed for the first appointment. Each subsequent appointment should build upon what is learned during this initial appointment and interview including:

- How much time is needed to effectively treat the patient?
- What will be accomplished at each visit?
- What accommodations will be necessary?
- How will success be measured?

Three brief 15-minute appointments can be scheduled with the patient, no more than 2 weeks apart, in order to maintain continuity and progression. The parent/caregiver should be encouraged to work on specific skills between visits. One way to consider billing each appointment is to charge for the exam on the first visit, fluoride varnish application at the second visit, and a prophylaxis at the third visit. Sequencing the appointments this way equals the same amount of chair time as an adult prophylaxis but allows the patient to return for more "short" successful visits. Any additional visits can use the ADA CDT 2011–2012 code for behavior management, D9920. This code is used by report in addition to treatment provided. It should be reported in 15-minute intervals (American Dental Association 2010).

Treating patients with developmental disorders involves effective communication skills and behavior guidance techniques as explained in earlier chapters. Depending on the patient's abilities, modifications in communication may be utilized. It is important to understand the patient's ability to understand language (receptive skill), as well as his or her ability to use language (expressive skill). Some patients may use an assistive communication device. Parents/caregivers should be encouraged to bring the device to all appointments. These communicative devices may be either electronic in nature or simple paper programs such as the Picture Exchange Communication System (PECS). PECS is a book with pictures that represent objects, people, places, and emotions that the patient is familiar with (DePalma & Raposa 2010). Patients with other types of communicative disorders may also benefit from PECS, and the dental practice can have a prepared book available for these patients. This will help in communicating the patient's wants and needs, along with assisting the dental professional in treatment outcomes.

The use of a reward system during treatment is an excellent motivation tool for patients with developmental disorders. Rewards strengthen the desired behaviors by enhancing their recurrence. Reward systems vary from patient to patient, and what enhances one patient's behavior may elicit a negative response from another. The dental professional needs to understand and use the appropriate reward system to enhance clinical treatments.

Distraction techniques for use during dental procedures are effective in assisting the dental professional during the treatment of a patient with a developmental disorder. Allowing the patient to take a short break (counting to a specific number) or singing and/or humming during procedures offers the patient the ability to remain in control, yet permits the dental professional to accomplish needed treatments. Other distraction techniques are discussed elsewhere in this text and can be valuable adjuncts to various procedures.

During the hygiene appointment itself, the goal is to provide consistent and predictable experiences for the patient. As dental professionals, creating an environment with reduced sensory stimuli, avoiding unnecessary touching, and utilizing four-handed dentistry as much as possible, while maintaining a high level of patience for repetition, can increase the success of treatments. The reinforcement of home care biofilm removal, scaling, and prophylaxis along with fluoride varnish applications can all occur during a successful hygiene appointment (Wilkins 2009). As with any patient, home care should be individualized, reinforced, and reevaluated at each visit. The differences are determined based on the patient's developmental age and life skills abilities. A patient who is unable to dress him- or herself or perform other self-help skills is unlikely to be able to perform oral hygiene independently. Many patients will require supervision and parental/caregiver involvement in their daily routines. The parent/caregiver can be provided with positioning technique options for home care procedures. One suggested document that illustrates some positioning options is *A Caregiver's Guide to Good Oral Health for Persons with Special Needs*, written by Dr. Steven Perlman, Dr. Clive Friedman, and Dr. Sanford Fenton. This booklet is available at www.specialolympics.org and can be downloaded and printed for distribution to families. The routine use of these positioning techniques at home can help prepare the patient for an examination or prophylaxis in the dental practice.

The use of protective stabilization devices during dental procedures is covered in depth in this textbook in Chapter 4. However, it is worth mentioning here that it is controversial and dental professionals need to consult their state dental practice acts regarding their usage (DePalma & Raposa 2010).

Reports indicate that persons with disabilities use tobacco products more than the general population (Rehabilitation Research and Training Center 2009). Therefore, tobacco use by patients and parents/caregivers should also be addressed during treatments and appropriate referrals and recommendations discussed.

Since many patients with developmental disorders are frequently given rewards that are food-based, dietary evaluations should also be part of the treatment discussions and appropriate recommendations provided. The use of remineralization products and full mouth disinfection will be discussed in detail in the next chapter and should also be suggested. The term "full mouth disinfection" is simply an alternative way of explaining oral hygiene, and it involves the change in vocabulary from the use of "toothpastes" and "toothbrushes" to the use of "medications" for the patient while the toothbrush becomes the "device" to deliver the medication. This is the perfect opportunity to help caregivers understand the importance of introducing a power toothbrush with an antibacterial toothpaste. There is a limited window of opportunity during the daily home care routine and using a power device with antibacterial toothpaste will provide the biggest benefit for the patient in the shortest amount of time. Changing the language of a message can raise the level of its importance. Reinforcement of any recommendations can be given to the patient, parent/caregiver in writing, or on the practice's Web site as appropriate. Furthermore, the integration of oral care routines into a child's individualized education program (IEP) can bridge the gap between home, school, and the dental practice. In addition, dental professionals can provide families with a prescription that states that the child should not receive sweet foods or excessive carbohydrates for rewards during school hours and this document can be placed in the individual's school record.

Each dental visit for the patient with a developmental disorder should build upon previous visits. Keeping instruments out of sight until needed, dividing the procedure or skill into smaller parts or segments, maintaining eye contact, and using educational modeling with clear, understandable directions—these allow patients and professionals to achieve success during treatments. Success is measured in the same manner as one measures success in general:

- How do the patient and parent/caregiver feel about visiting the dental practice?
- How does the patient respond to treatment?
- Evaluation of actual home care routines.
- Presence/absence of new disease.
- Documentation of successes and failures (DePalma & Raposa 2009).

After the initial appointment and following any future appointments, a member of the dental team who cared for the patient should consider a follow-up phone call or e-mail as appropriate. By providing a follow-up contact, the practice reinforces its commitment to the patient and/or parent/caregiver and helps the patient and the family by becoming an advocate and champion toward positive results. Depending on the procedure performed or procedures recommended at home, the contact can be the next day or a week later to provide positive reinforcement. Providing this support to those involved can increase the success rates of further treatments and recommendations.

The long-term impact of successful dental treatment can provide lifelong dental health for patients with a developmental disorder. It demonstrates that there are others who care for them and allows them the ability to focus on one less stressful event. For the family of the patient with a developmental disorder, the impact can provide the feeling of acceptance where others have not and an increase in trust that will translate into positive word-of-mouth statements about the practice. For the practice, the impact of treating the patient with a developmental disorder can be realized by experiencing an increase in referrals, hearing that the team has a reputation for being caring, thoughtful, and kind; and experiencing opportunities to meet and help a group of wonderful families. On a personal level, the experience is one that can bring immeasurable rewards and elation by providing the opportunities to impact a patient or family in a major way. "To the world, you might just be one person, but to one person you just might be the world" (John H. MacDonald, Jr.).

## REFERENCES

American Dental Association. (2010). *CDT 2011–2012, ADA Practical Guide to Dental Procedure Codes.*

DePalma AM, Raposa K. (2009). *Building Bridges: Dental Care for Patients with Autism.* Tulsa: PennWell Publishing.

———. (2010). *Understanding and Guiding the Dental Patient with Autism,* Part 2. Tulsa: PennWell Publishing.

Rehabilitation Research and Training Center on Disability Statistics and Demographics. (2009). Annual Disability Statistics Compendium.

Wilkins E. (2009). *Clinical Practice of the Dental Hygienist,* 10th ed. Baltimore: Lippincott Williams & Wilkins.

# Preventing oral health problems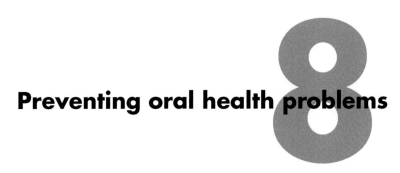

Paul Glassman, DDS, MA, MBA and
Christine E. Miller, RDH, MHS, MA

## INTRODUCTION

In most respects preventing oral diseases among people with disabilities involves using the same strategies that are employed with other segments of the population. However, there are a number of unique factors that make preventing oral diseases among people with disabilities more complex than with other segments of the population and require additional strategies to be successful. These include the following:

- People with cognitive impairments may not understand the importance of having a healthy mouth or what needs to be done to have a healthy mouth.
- People with physical limitations may not be able to perform needed procedures.
- Some people may be resistive to performing mouth care procedures or to having someone else help them or perform these procedures for them.
- Some people with disabilities have primary or associated medical problems that increase their risk for having poor oral health. Among other things, they may take one or more of the more than 400 medications that cause xerostomia (Oral Biotech 2011; Turner & Ship 2007).
- Many people with disabilities are dependent on others for activities of daily living, including mouth care activities. Some caregivers have

*Treating the Dental Patient with a Developmental Disorder*, First Edition.
Edited by Karen A. Raposa and Steven P. Perlman.
© 2012 John Wiley & Sons, Inc. Published 2012 by John Wiley & Sons, Inc.

limited understanding about the causes of oral diseases or methods to care for their own mouth, let alone the mouth of the person they are caring for. Even when caregivers value prevention and know how to perform preventive procedures, it is more complex for oral health professionals to help prevent oral diseases when there is a third party involved.

In addition to the challenges faced by people with disabilities or their caregivers with understanding and performing preventive procedures, many people with disabilities have more dental disease and more difficulty obtaining dental care than other segments of the population (U.S. Department of Health and Human Services 2000; Oral Health America 2000; Haavio 1995; Feldman et al. 1997; Waldman et al. 2000; United States General Accounting Office 2000; Glassman & Miller 2003; Cohen et al. 2011).

## OVERCOMING OBSTACLES TO ORAL HEALTH

The authors have developed a set of training and organizational materials over the past several decades to address the challenges in improving and maintaining oral health for people with special needs. The materials, called *Overcoming Obstacles to Oral Health*, are currently in their 5th edition (Glassman et al. 2011). The materials address obstacles to oral health in four areas. These four areas should be the focus of any program to maintain oral health for people with disabilities. They are:

- Overcoming information obstacles—does the individual or his or her caregivers understand what needs to be done?
- Overcoming physical obstacles—can the individual or his or her caregivers physically perform needed procedures?
- Overcoming behavioral obstacles—is the individual resistant to performing or having someone else perform preventive procedures?
- Overcoming organizational obstacles—is there a system in the home, community, or facility where the individual resides that can support and help his or her caregivers and the individual overcome the other three obstacles?

## OVERCOMING INFORMATION OBSTACLES

The first area to assess when working with an individual or caregiver is the person's level of understanding about the value of good oral health, the causes and consequences of poor oral health, and the procedures to perform to maintain good oral health. When making such an assessment, it is important to consider the setting and strategies for assessing the level of knowledge and conveying new information. Issues such as socio-economic status, race, ethnicity, age, gender, native language, cultural beliefs, how the individual best receives health information, and the best setting for delivering information are important to understand and incorporate in any group or individual oral health literacy assessment or improvement efforts (Institute of Medicine 2011). In many circumstances providing the traditional short lesson on "oral hygiene" or even a longer "anticipatory guidance" session delivered at the end of a dental appointment in a dental office may not have any impact on the subsequent behavior of the individual or his or her caregivers (American Academy of Pediatric Dentistry 2009; Glassman & Miller 2006). For some individuals effective health promotion messages may best be delivered in a community setting such as the individual's residence, a school, a work program, or a location where the person receives other social or general health services. It is critical that oral health professionals who work in dental offices and clinics recognize the limitations of delivering oral health messages in the dental office setting and the value of partnering with community-based resources. A separate chapter in this book describes the importance and use of community-based systems of care.

Whatever the circumstances where oral health messages are delivered, it is important to do so using simple language, referring to pictures and simple diagrams whenever possible, delivering small amounts of information at any one time, testing understanding, repeating information and adding new information at subsequent sessions, and creating an environment where individuals or caregivers feel comfortable asking questions.[15] Even more significant than delivering messages in the optimum time and place and using the message delivery strategies described above is the ability to tailor the message to the beliefs and values of the person being addressed. For example, *motivational interviewing* is a technique for understanding the beliefs and values of the individual and customizing oral health strategies to help the individual achieve his or her own goals. This method has been shown to result in greater improvement in oral health than traditional health education (Weinstein et al. 2006).

In addition to understanding the best strategies for delivering oral health information, it is also important to understand that providing information, even when it results in knowledge increase, does not necessarily lead to behavior change (Freeman & Ismail 2009; Satur et al. 2010). In fact, a 2000 report by the Institute of Medicine on social and behavioral research stated that "To prevent disease, we increasingly ask people to do things that they have not done previously, to stop doing things they have been doing for years, and to do more of some things and less of other things. Although there certainly are examples of successful programs to change behavior, it is clear that behavior change is a difficult and complex challenge. It is unreasonable to expect that people will change their behavior easily when so many forces in the social, cultural, and physical environment conspire against such change" (Institute of Medicine

2000). In fact, in a study published in 2006, Glassman and Miller demonstrated that caregiver knowledge about preventive procedures was improved after training, but this was only translated into behavior change with incorporation of new techniques into daily routines after a dental assistant observed the prevention session in the residential environment and provided hands-on, real-time coaching (Glassman & Miller 2006).

The next consideration in overcoming information obstacles is deciding what information to provide. The authors recommend starting with the benefits of performing oral health preventive procedures. Particularly when working with caregivers it is critical that they understand why improving the oral health of the person they are supporting is beneficial to the caregivers themselves. Benefits for caregivers can include reduced mouth odors, making it more pleasant to be with the person; reduced acting-out behaviors, making it easier to work with the person; people who are more interactive with others; people who can eat without mouth pain and require less care; and pride among caregivers at seeing the people they work with become healthier with a happier smile.

Once the individual or caregiver understands the benefits of improved oral health for themselves and the person they care for, then they are more likely to be open to receiving additional information. At this point they can be provided with information about the difference between a healthy mouth and an unhealthy one, how to recognize oral health problems, and how to perform plaque removal techniques. These topics are all illustrated in the *Overcoming Obstacles to Oral Health* training materials described earlier (Glassman et al. 2011).

It is also important that any preventive program include an assessment of the individual's risk for developing oral diseases and the use of a customized regimen of preventive medications. The *Caries Management by Risk Assessment* (CAMBRA) model is a system for determining risk of dental caries and providing targeted medications to alter the chemistry and environment of the mouth (Young et al. 2007). Particularly for dependent people, where it can be difficult to treat dental disease once it occurs, it is critical that prevention protocols include modern "medical" strategies incorporating medications such as fluoride in various forms, chlorhexidine, xylitol, buffering agents, and calcium phosphate replacement agents (Glassman 2003; Glassman et al. 2003). A detailed discussion of the indications for and use of these medications is beyond the scope of this chapter.

Finally, it is important when working with individuals or caregivers of individuals who live in group settings to make sure they understand proper infection control procedures to follow when performing preventive procedures and when using and storing oral hygiene implements. It may be surprising to some oral health professionals, but it should not be assumed that caregivers in group residential settings understand the risks involved in exposing themselves or other residents to potentially infectious agents or understand techniques for using or storing mouth care supplies that will prevent the spread of infectious agents.

## OVERCOMING PHYSICAL OBSTACLES

Another barrier to prevention of dental disease is physical. Some people understand what needs to be done but lack the musculature, dexterity, or coordination to do it. There are numerous adaptations and aids that can help overcome these physical barriers. Figure 8.1 shows toothbrushes that have been adapted with a larger handle using a tennis ball or bicycle handle grip. Figure 8.2 shows someone with limited dexterity using a large foam ball as a means of picking up a toothbrush. Similar adaptation can be made for floss holders.

A general principle in working with people with special needs is that they should be encouraged to do as much as possible for themselves. However, if they have limited ability to perform daily mouth care procedures, they may need help from a caregiver to complete these procedures. This is referred to as "partial participation." Many caregivers try to brush someone's teeth or perform other procedures while standing behind the person in the bathroom. In this position they have difficulty seeing, have to stop frequently to allow the individual to spit, and generally cannot effectively perform the needed procedures. It is useful to realize that, although most people remove plaque and apply fluoride in the form of fluoride toothpaste at the same time, it is not necessary to do it that way. If the caregiver will first remove plaque with only a damp toothbrush and then later apply fluoride toothpaste, the caregiver will have increased freedom to perform mouth care activities outside of the bathroom in a location where he or she can see and be effective.

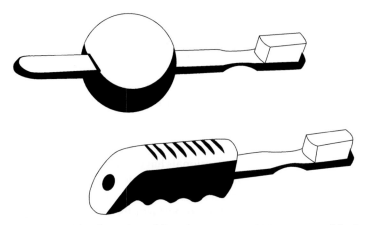

**Figure 8.1**   Toothbrushes adapted for easier grip. © 1998 University of the Pacific School of Dentistry Department of Dental Practice and Community Services. Reprinted with permission.

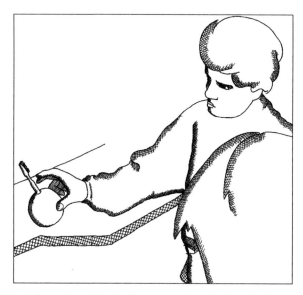

**Figure 8.2**    Adapted toothbrush for someone with limited dexterity. © 1998 University of the Pacific School of Dentistry Department of Dental Practice and Community Services. Reprinted with permission.

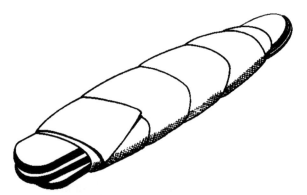

**Figure 8.3**    A tongue blade mouth rest. © 1998 University of the Pacific School of Dentistry Department of Dental Practice and Community Services. Reprinted with permission.

Oral health professionals have an important role in teaching caregivers who are helping someone complete daily mouth care procedures how to position the person and themselves so they can have the best visibility possible and be able to perform the needed procedures as thoroughly and easily as possible. There are several positioning techniques that can make it easier for a caregiver to help someone complete daily mouth care procedures. Figure 8.3 is an illustration of a disposable "tongue blade

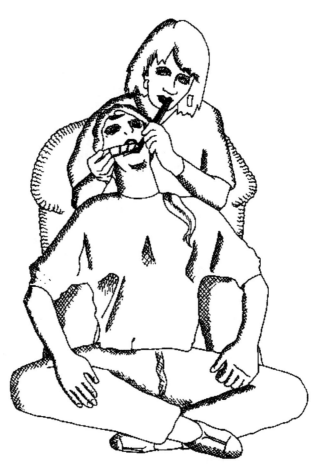

**Figure 8.4** Partial participation, using positioning and a mouth rest. © 1998 University of the Pacific School of Dentistry Department of Dental Practice and Community Services. Reprinted with permission.

mouth rest." This type of mouth rest can be easily constructed by a caregiver from readily available materials and can be very useful in helping someone complete daily mouth care procedures. There are also commercially available disposable and reusable mouth rests (Specialized Care Co., Inc. 2011).

Figure 8.4 shows the use of a mouth rest with someone who is sitting on the floor with the head resting on the caregiver's shoulders. Note the use of the forefingers of the left and right hand in stabilizing the head. Figure 8.5 again shows the use of a mouth rest. This time the individual may be less able to help and is positioned on a couch. Note the use of the right forearm and the tongue blade in stabilizing the head. These positions allow the caregiver to see and gain access to parts of the mouth that would be difficult in other positions. Dental professionals can play a pivotal role

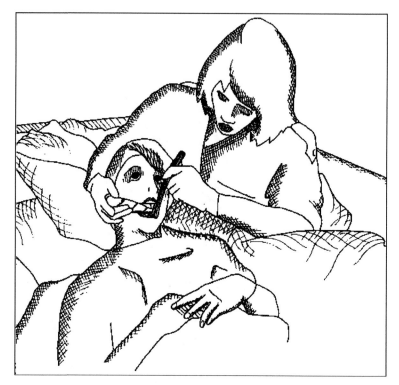

**Figure 8.5**   Partial participation, using positioning and a mouth rest. © 1998 University of the Pacific School of Dentistry Department of Dental Practice and Community Services. Reprinted with permission.

in educating caregivers about the benefits and use of physical adaptations and partial participation.

## OVERCOMING BEHAVIORAL OBSTACLES

Some people are resistant to performing daily mouth care activities or having someone help them. This may be due to limited ability to understand what is being asked or to cooperate as a result of intellectually disability, cognitive impairment from other causes, or tactile sensitivity. There are numerous guidelines and techniques that are available to help caregivers work with such individuals, reduce resistive behaviors, and gain cooperation (Lyons 2009; American Academy of Pediatric Dentistry 2008). Earlier terminology referred to "behavior management" techniques. This terminology is now being replaced by terminology like "behavior support." Although the guidelines just referenced and many others like them are written for a professional audience, there are simple principles that can be taught to caregivers and adapted for individual situations. The *Overcoming Obstacles to Oral Health* training materials referred to earlier provide specific training for caregivers on using behavioral support strategies to improve cooperation with resistive people (Glassman et al. 2011).

There are several basic principles that can be taught to caregivers for reducing resistive behavior that will be briefly described here. These are:

- Structuring the environment—this refers to picking a place or time of day that is more conducive to gaining cooperation than other times or places. It may be a place or time that reduces distractions, removes unpleasant associations to mouth care procedures, or makes mouth care procedures seem fun.
- Involving the individual—some people with disabilities, especially those who reside in group living or institutional living arrangements, may have very regimented lives. They may be told when to wake up, when to eat, when to use the bathroom, what to wear, and what they will do during the day. Anything that a caregiver can do to increase choices can aid cooperation. This can be as simple as being able to choose when to brush one's teeth or what color a new toothbrush will be. It also involves paying attention to how someone is doing and not pushing the person so far that a pleasant mouth care session turns into an unpleasant one.
- Using reinforcers—we all respond to things that are rewarding to us by wanting to continue or increase the activity that produced the reward. When carefully selected and applied, rewards can motivate people to become more and more independent in daily mouth care practices. It is important to use things that are actually rewarding for the individual, to monitor the effect of the reward over time, and to change it if necessary. Caregivers can be educated to realize that social rewards, like smiling and praise, can be as powerful for people with disabilities as they are for everyone else.
- Shaping—shaping is the reinforcement of an action that is an approximation of the task. If you would like someone to brush for 5 minutes, you might use a reinforcer after 30 seconds at first. Later the reinforcer might not be used until 1 or 2 minutes have passed. It is also critical to make sure that each session is a pleasant one and ends with the individual having a good feeling about him- or herself and oral health activities.
- Simple and direct communication techniques—some people have trouble hearing or seeing well or may not understand verbal communication very well. Some simple and direct techniques that caregivers can use to improve communication include:
  - Establish eye contact.
  - Use simple declarative sentences.
  - Use words and phrases that are perceived as helping, not giving orders.
  - Speak in a calm but friendly and firm voice using the individual's name frequently.

○ Give one instruction at a time.

○ Offer choices whenever possible.

These techniques are often combined into a "desensitization" process where slow, gradual progress is made toward a goal. Oral health professionals can be instrumental in helping a caregiver design and carry out a plan for desensitization that results in gradual improvement in cooperation for daily mouth care.

## OVERCOMING ORGANIZATIONAL OBSTACLES

Many people with disabilities live in group settings. These settings can include group home or residential facilities or institutions that provide some level of health care services (Glassman & Subar 2010). In these settings there are often organizational policies and structures that impact how daily mouth care activities are performed. Oral health professionals can significantly improve oral health of individuals living in these group settings by working with the leaders of the facility to establish an oral health program that becomes integrated into the policies and structures of the organization (Glassman et al. 2011). Some characteristics of an effective oral health program are:

- Oral health becomes incorporated into the mission of the facility so everyone knows that maintaining oral health for the residents of the facility is a core value and practice.
- The top leaders in the facility communicate to everyone associated with the facility that oral health is important and good oral health is an expectation for all residents.
- The top leaders in the facility help communicate the importance and benefits for everyone in the facility of the residents having good oral health.
- Training, coaching, and mentoring for direct care staff is provided to help them perform effective daily mouth care for the facility's residents.
- There is a system for supervision, monitoring, and rewarding direct care staff to ensure that they perform effective daily mouth care for the facility's residents.
- There is a system for purchasing, inventorying, and providing mouth care products that are needed as a part of the oral health program.

Working with, training, and supporting leaders in residential facilities may not be the usual techniques that oral health professionals use in an office-based practice. Oral health professionals may need to expand their vision of their professional role and responsibility to take on this type of activity. However, those who do this will be rewarded by seeing their patients improve their ability to maintain their oral health and require fewer complex dental procedures.

# PUTTING IT ALL TOGETHER

Many of the principles discussed in this chapter may be new to oral health professionals or to people with disabilities or their caregivers. An effective method to help people with disabilities or their caregivers remember the techniques or steps to good mouth health is to write them down in a plan. A written plan makes it easier to remember what needs to be done, communicate the plan to others who may be involved, and check whether the plan is being carried out. The *Overcoming Obstacles to Oral Health* training materials contain an example of a "Daily Mouth Care Plan" (Glassman et al. 2011). That plan includes the following sections:

- Assessment—what is the problem that needs to be addressed now? What techniques should be taught or applied to the problem at this time?
- Tools and products—what tools can help with daily mouth care now? Examples include adapted or special brushes or plaque removal tools, partial participation positioning, mouth rests, or medications.
- Physical/behavior plan—what techniques are being used now to reduce resistive behavior? These include a description of the ability of the individual, what can be expected of the person now, what conditions can best lead to success, if is there is a desensitization program in place and if so, what steps and rewards are being used.
- Professional dental care plan—what is the plan for upcoming or periodic professional dental care?

All the techniques described in this chapter sound separate. However, as oral health professionals work with individuals with disabilities, their caregivers, or leaders in the residences or facilities where they live, they can be combined into an effective strategy that can improve oral health and reduce the development of further dental disease. Oral health professionals have a great opportunity to expand the prevention techniques they use and make an important difference in the oral health and lives of people with disabilities.

# REFERENCES

American Academy of Pediatric Dentistry. (2008). Guideline on behavior guidance for the pediatric dental patient.

———. (2009). Guideline on periodicity of examination, preventive dental services, anticipatory guidance/counseling, and oral treatment for infants, children, and adolescents.

Cohen LA, Bonito AJ, Eicheldinger C, et al. (2011). Behavioral and socioeconomic correlates of dental problem experience and patterns of health care-seeking. *Journal of the American Dental Association* 142:137–149.

Feldman CA, Giniger M, Sanders M, Saporito R, Zohn HK, Perlman SP. (1997). Special Olympics, Special Smiles: Assessing the feasibility of epidemiologic data collection. *Journal of the American Dental Association* 128:1687–1696.

Freeman R, Ismail A. (2009). Assessing patients' health behaviours: Essential steps for motivating patients to adopt and maintain behaviours conducive to oral health. *Monographs in Oral Science* 21:113–127.

Glassman P. (2003). Practical protocols for the prevention of dental disease in community settings for people with special needs: Preface. *Special Care in Dentistry* 23(5):157–159.

Glassman P, et al. (2003). Practical protocols for the prevention of dental disease in community settings for people with special needs: The protocols. *Special Care in Dentistry* 23(5):160–164.

Glassman P, Miller C. (2003). Preventing dental disease for people with special needs: The need for practical preventive protocols for use in community settings. *Special Care in Dentistry* 23(5):165–167.

——— . (2006). Effect of preventive dentistry training program for caregivers in community facilities on caregiver and client behavior and client oral hygiene. *New York State Dental Journal* 72(2):38–46.

Glassman P, Miller C, Helgeson M, et al. (2011). *Overcoming Obstacles to Oral Health: A Training Program for Caregivers of People with Disabilities and Frail Elders*, 5th ed. Accessed June 19, 2011, from http://www.dental.pacific.edu/ Community_Involvement/Pacific_Center_for_Special_Care_(PCSC)/ Special_Care_Resources/Overcoming_Obstacles.html.

Glassman P, Miller C, Wozniak T, Jones C. (1994). A preventive dentistry training program for persons with disabilities residing in community residential facilities. *Special Care in Dentistry* 14(4):137–143.

Glassman P, Subar P. (2010). Creating and maintaining oral health for dependent people in institutional settings. *Journal of Public Health Dentistry* 70:S40–S48.

Haavio ML. (1995). Oral health care of the mentally retarded and other persons with disabilities in the Nordic countries: Present situation and plans for the future. *Special Care in Dentistry* 15:65–69.

Institute of Medicine. (2000). *Promoting Health: Intervention Strategies from Social and Behavioral Research*. Washington, DC: National Academies Press.

——— . (2011). *Advancing Oral Health in America*. Washington D.C.: National Academies Press.

Lyons R. (2009). Understanding basic behavioral support techniques as an alternative to sedation and anesthesia. *Special Care in Dentistry* 29(1):39–50.

Miller C, Glassman P. (1995). Beyond brushing: Training dental students to assess and create oral health plans for people with disabilities. *Journal of Dental Education* 59(2):133 (abstract).

Oral Biotech. (2011). Medications that may cause dry mouth. Accessed June 19, 2011, from http://www.carifree.com/media/Dry%20Mouth%20Medications.pdf.

Oral Health America. (2000). The disparity cavity: Filling America's oral health gap.

Satur JG, Gussy MG, Morgan MV, Calache H, Wright C. (2010). Review of the evidence for oral health promotion effectiveness. *Health Education Journal* 69(3):257–266.

Specialized Care Co., Inc. (2011). Open Wide Mouth Rests. Accessed June 15, 2011, from http://www.specializedcare.com/shop/pc/viewCategories.asp?idCategory=18.

Turner MD, Ship JA. (2007). Dry mouth and its effects on the oral health of elderly people. *Journal of the American Dental Association* 138(9 supplement):15S–20S.

U.S. Department of Health and Human Services. (2000). Oral health in America: A report of the Surgeon General. Rockville, MD: U.S. Department of Health and Human Services, National Institute of Dental and Craniofacial Research, National Institutes of Health.

U.S. General Accounting Office. (2000). Oral health: Factors contributing to low use of dental services by low-income populations. Report to Congressional Requesters.

Waldman HB, Perlman SP, Swerdloff M. (2000). Use of pediatric dental services in the 1990s: Some continuing difficulties. *Journal of Dentistry for Children* 67:59–63.

Weinstein P, Harrison R, Benton T. (2006). Motivating mothers to prevent caries: Confirming the beneficial effect of counseling. *Journal of the American Dental Association* 137:789–793.

Young D, Featherstone J, Roth J. (2007). Caries management by risk assessment: A practitioner's guide. *CDA Journal* 35(10):679–680.

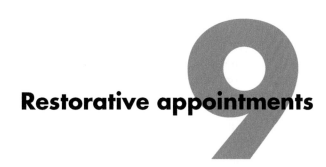

# Restorative appointments

Federico Garcia-Godoy, DDS, MA and
Cristina E. Garcia-Godoy, DDS, CCRP, MPH

People with developmental disabilities/disorders (DDDs) generally present with increased oral health problems compared to the general population. For this reason, it is important to focus on each patient's specific needs in order to achieve optimal oral health. No two persons are alike, not even twins! It is extremely important to keep this in mind, especially when treating individuals with DDDs. Improving the oral health of a person with DDDs may be slow at first, but determination and communication can bring positive results.

Unfortunately, most academic programs in dental schools worldwide advocate the use of general anesthesia for patients with DDDs and fail to consider behavior management/guidance as a viable option when treating these individuals. General and pediatric dentistry programs have shifted from a clinic-based operation to more of a hospital-based perspective, referring patients with DDDs directly to the hospital's operating room without assessing the behavioral situation, therefore increasing barriers to a more appropriate treatment: behavior management/guidance.

## SETTING UP FOR SUCCESS

Providing oral health care services to patients with DDDs requires an adjustment of our everyday skills, as some DDDs such as autism spectrum disorders (ASDs), cerebral palsy, Down syndrome, and intellectual

*Treating the Dental Patient with a Developmental Disorder*, First Edition.
Edited by Karen A. Raposa and Steven P. Perlman.
© 2012 John Wiley & Sons, Inc. Published 2012 by John Wiley & Sons, Inc.

disabilities (IDs) can affect the mind, the body, and the skills of thinking, talking, and self-care. Those inflicted need extra help to achieve and maintain good oral health. It has been established that those with chronic medical illnesses, developmental disabilities, and psychosocial issues experience more oral health care problems than others who do not suffer from these conditions (Havio 1995; Feldman et al. 1997; Waldman et al. 2000).

Knowing the background of your target population, in this case DDDs, will enhance your possibilities of success in presenting an adequate treatment plan and subsequent successful restorative appointments. The dental team may be inattentive to communication styles, but the patient and his or her parents are not (Hall et al. 1987). These relationship and communications problems have been shown to play a prominent role in initiating malpractice actions (Lester & Smith 1993).

## STRATEGIES FOR CARE

The optimum development of correct attitudes will give us a correct approach to an effective dental restorative treatment for patients with DDDs.

### Knowing your patient's developmental disability/disorder

Before the restorative appointment, make sure you have reviewed DDDs and the different manifestations and possible complications. Consult the patient's physician, family, or caregivers to achieve an accurate medical/dental history. Specific questions regarding the disability of the patient will provide valuable information about the patient's level of function and will help us identify the patient's support system. The disability may require adjustment of the patient's position in the dental chair, as those individuals with congestive heart failure, asthma, high-level spinal cord injuries, cerebral palsy, and/or swallowing difficulties will require a more upright position.

To properly treat patients with DDDs and, if necessary, refer them for appropriate medical care, dental professionals must be able to recognize the signs and symptoms of each patient's specific disability (Raposa 2009).

Medications used to treat cardiovascular, psychiatric, chronic respiration, and other disorders may interact with dental agents, including anesthetics, vasoconstrictors, and sedatives; therefore these agents may be avoided or used with extreme caution and medical supervision.

Most people with DDDs can be treated successfully in the general practice setting with few procedural alterations. It is important to introduce the patient to the staff and setting before placing him or her in a hospital operating room. If placed immediately, it will only indicate, in our opinion, a clear refusal of treatment. There is no need for a specialty degree to perform operative work on a patient who is sleeping and controlled; some knowledge of general anesthesia and the hospital setting protocols will suffice.

In the 30-year clinical and academic practice of one of the authors of this chapter (FGG), general anesthesia has been used for only very profound cases of patients with DDDs. Behavioral techniques have generally proved adequate in the dental office and university environment. Transferring these patients to the hospital environment risks the "labeling" of patients with DDDs. Complete knowledge of the condition and effective communication will enhance your approach toward patients with DDDs.

During assessment, the dentist should consider not only the physical/medical risk for the individual but also social issues, which could help enhance patient as well as parent/caregiver satisfaction (Girdler & Hill 1988). Patient satisfaction, both during treatment and after care, is an important goal, and patients by right should have their concerns about care taken into account (Baker 1990).

## Treatment planning

The ideal components of an accurate treatment plan in patients with DDDs have to include (Figure 9.1):

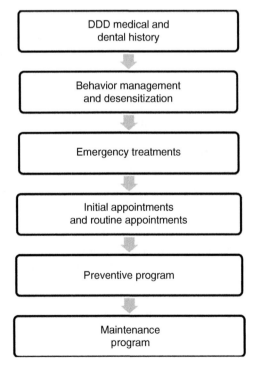

**Figure 9.1**    Ideal components of an accurate treatment plan for patients with developmental disabilities/disorders.

a.  *DDD medical and dental history*—it is necessary to understand the meaning of all signs and symptoms of the different DDDs, as well as the dental history. This will provide a complete picture of the patient's needs so that proper intervention may be achieved.

b.  *Behavior guidance and desensitization*—behavior guidance techniques are an important tool for success. Understanding a variety of ways to guide the patient will help accomplish a smooth and workable rapport. Behavior guidance techniques are covered in more detail in Chapter 4.

c.  *Emergency care strategies*—the first phase of any treatment plan is to address the cause of pain and acute infection. Dental emergencies that can affect the quality of life in patients with DDDs are medical emergencies. These include cardiovascular events, seizures, choking, and allergic reactions, which are caused most frequently by the interaction of medication and dental agents (e.g., local anesthesia). The dental team should know how to handle the events and stay current with procedures and cautions. These procedures should be readily accessible and clearly written for the dental staff.

Potential dental or medical emergencies should be considered before any other dental treatment is considered.

Dental urgencies differ from dental emergencies in that they do not require immediate attention and are generally noted during routine patient examination (e.g., asymptomatic deep carious lesion).

The following can be considered as dental emergencies (Abbud et al. 2002; Mani et al. 1997):

1.  Jaw and/or alveolar bone fractures.
2.  Avulsed or displaced teeth.
3.  Fractured teeth with pulp exposure.
4.  Acute alveolar abscess.
5.  Upper airway impairment.
6.  Oral mucosa lacerations.
7.  Acute dental pain.
8.  Uncontrolled bleeding.

Dentists who provide sedation service in their dental office should have the ADA documents and guidelines readily available (ADA 2000).

Determining medical conditions associated with aberrant behavior in patients with DDDs could be difficult. Effective communication will help ease this identification problem.

Pyles et al. (1997) described three very important ways to interpret some abnormal behavior:

1.  *Physical discomfort or illness*—are more likely to snap at others or act in ways they normally do not. Hormonal changes (menstruation) can exacerbate frustrating or adverse events.

2. *Pain or discomfort*—escape-motivated behavior; diving out of the wheel-chair after prolonged sitting; refusing to eat because of dental problem.
3. *Communication deficits*   maladaptive behavior may be the only way that patients with DDDs can alert others of a problem (e.g., when he or she is wet, has an earache, or is hungry).

d. *Introducing dental care services (time for the organization of the initial appointments and routine appointments)*—once the information regarding the patient, including the DDD history and the medical/dental history, is collected, care services can be initiated. Behavior management strategies can then be tailored before the first appointment. Informed consents will be obtained from the parent/guardian.

e. *Initial appointment and interview*—this component of the treatment plan describes surgical and restorative work planned to address the individual's dental needs and to determine how these procedures will be performed. It is also the time to confirm medical and DDD history obtained prior to the patient's visit. In the prior meeting with parent/guardian/caregiver, ask if you should make any special arrrangements in advance; an interpreter, for example, may be required if the patient has hearing loss or is not able to speak or communicate. Federal laws prohibit discrimination against persons with disabilities and require hospitals to provide "effective communication" for persons who are deaf or hard of hearing (National Association of the Deaf 1990).

f. *Preventive program*—once the multifactorial behavior of the carious disease has been clearly observed, it is important to establish a preventive program (Figure 9.2) that accomplishes the identification of the close and active relationship among the professional determinants, the socio-economic determinants, the biological determinants, and the biofilm of the tooth structure (Garcia-Godoy 2009).

g. *Maintenance programs*—a careful and well–planned maintenance program has to be established according to the patient's personal needs in order to ensure proper routine appointments.

# RESTORATIVE TREATMENTS

## Strategies for operatory procedures and biomaterials

Restorative treatments in patients with DDDs immediately uncover three issues that are the primary concerns of the clinician:

- Use of local anesthesia.
- Use of rubber dam.
- What is the best restorative material?

One of the issues that arises concerning the use of *local anesthesia* in patients with DDDs is lip biting. We have not seen any surprising adverse

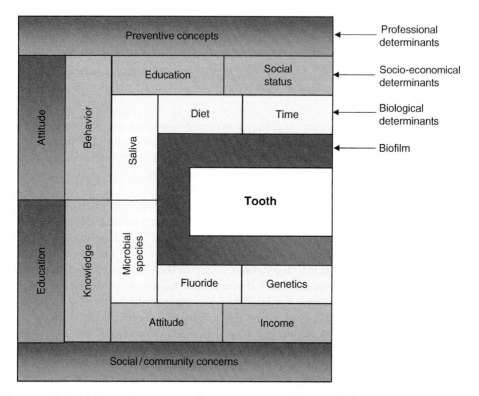

**Figure 9.2**   Multifactorial interaction of caries components (Garcia-Godoy 2009).

effects during regular dental treatments. When caries spots or infections are not deep or pulp-involving, we do not use local anesthesia in our patients with or without a DDD. When a patient is well oriented by behavior management/guidance, its use can be alleviated. When needed, a local anesthetic may be used with a shorter needle, which is less likely to bend or break.

Another issue that arises is the use of the *rubber dam* for restorative procedures. While we agree with the positive benefits of the use of the rubber dam, we also understand that the effectiveness is increased with cooperative patients but decreased when a patient is uncooperative or has uncontrolled movements and limited understanding, as is the case with many of the patients with DDD. The rubber dam is typically very difficult to place, and the necessity for securing the clamp becomes increasingly important.

We must also remember that certain DDD patients are mouth breathers, which may cause undue anxiety over airway obstruction when the dam is used.

A local anesthetic, combined when possible with behavior management/guidance techniques, remains the approach of choice unless there is a need to carry out multiple operatory procedures in one session, in which case we may choose conscious sedation techniques.

As we have mentioned before, with certain accommodations, patients with DDD can generally be successfully treated in the dental office environment. Operatory procedures are the most common of our "treatment" approaches, and this of course, as in all areas of dentistry, has been bringing up issues regarding different materials used for restorations in patients with DDDs.

Previously, *dental amalgam* has been pointed out as the "bad guy" because of its mercury "association" with neurological functions of certain developmental disabilities/disorders. It has been reported that mercury levels in autopsy tissue from fetuses and infants correlate with the number of dental amalgams in the mother (Drasch et al. 1994). Vapors escaping into the oral cavity during the placement or removal of amalgam restorations, once inhaled, travel through the placenta, representing a potential source of exposure to the fetus (Davidson et al. 2004). Harada (1968) documented twenty-two cases of congenital Minamata disease in pregnant women who consumed contaminated fish with high levels of methyl mercury (MeHg). The mothers manifested mild or no symptoms but gave birth to infants with severe developmental disabilities, including cerebral palsy, intellectual disability, and seizures. This was followed by several studies in different countries showing similar reports (Marsh et al. 1995; Mckeown-Eyssen et al. 1983; Kjellstrom et al. 1989; Ramirez et al. 2000; Grandjean et al. 1999). An association between amalgam exposure and neurological signs of clinically evident peripheral neuropathy was not found by some authors (Kingsman et al. 2005; Bellinger et al. 2007a, 2007b; Lauterbach et al. 2008; Bellinger et al. 2008; Bates et al. 2004; Ye et al. 2009).

On the other hand, mercury levels have been detected as low in amniotic fluid with no negative reactions during pregnancy, such as hypertension, rupture of membrane, caesarean section rate, miscarriage, or postpartum hemorrhage. Likewise, hypocalcaemia, hypoglycemia, hyperbilirubinemia, sepsis, respiratory distress syndrome, asphyxia, and seizure were not seen in the newborns (Luglie et al. 2005; Palkovicova et al. 2008; Hujoel et al. 2005; Daniels et al. 2007; Geier et al. 2009; Lindbohm et al. 2007; da Costa et al. 2005).

For some clinicians, amalgam remains the primary choice of restorative material for the disabled patient primarily due to the belief that it is less technique sensitive, especially where a dry field is impossible to obtain. We, on the other hand, discarded dental amalgam from our practice almost 15 years ago, for both technical and ecological reasons. We have found that new materials, if used according to the manufacturer's recommendations, show the best results both technically and aesthetically.

From a technical point of view, amalgam restorations require a more extensive cavity for support and may be more susceptible to fracture. Newer marketed materials offer great opportunities for restorative procedures on patients with DDDs, satisfying their dental needs as well as elevating the self-esteem of the patient through a better aesthetic result. Placement of amalgam restorations requires reasonable access to the cavity preparation for lengthy periods of time in order to adequately condense without contamination.

*Polyacid-modified resin composites* (compomers) may present similar problems in placement of the material. In the presence of a high caries rate these will not be the material of choice due to the lack of resistance to accumulation of bacterial plaque (Smith & Williams 1982). The mechanical adhesion with enamel is dependent upon the presence of sound, well-mineralized enamel, which may be hard to find (Gryst & Mount 1999). Composite resin is the best choice when aesthetics is of consideration. It can be used in fractures in anterior teeth, when a cast restoration is impossible. It can be constructed with autopolymerized or light-cured composite utilizing a clear crown former, or manually. Occlusion is of great importance to avoid fractures. In these cases (anterior restorations) we can construct the crown shorter than usual to avoid contact and further reduce the possibility of fracture. Ellis et al. (1992) described the indirect fabrication of composite resin crowns for the primary anterior teeth. We have used this technique treating ectodermal dysplasia, baby-bottle caries, and fractures in patients with DDDs. The technique indeed reduces clinical time, provides a durable restoration, and allows treatment for those who will not withstand a long procedure. We do not use composite resins in the posterior region due to the technique sensitive condition.

At this point we have to remember that we need a personal approach to each patient. The "ideal" patient, the one we see in the textbooks and even sometimes in the dental office, is not the general rule. With behavior-disrupted patients or patients with DDDs, the approach has to be modified and individualized, according to the patient's needs.

Some patients with DDDs can be perfect candidates for long treatment appointments where you can use the rubber dam, composite resins, and even multiple restorations in one single appointment. Others will require your patience and training and probably more time to accomplish the treatment plan and less time for the restorative appointments. This makes the proper selection of materials very important.

*Glass ionomer* is our material of choice for patients with DDDs because the advantages include adhesion to both enamel and dentin (Mount 1989) and a continuous fluoride release, apparently sufficient to reduce or inhibit plaque buildup (Forsten 1994). Glass ionomers are simple and easy to handle under difficult circumstances and "tolerant" to placement in a humid atmosphere over mildly wet dentin because, as water-based cements, they require a degree of humidity to maintain the water balance during setting (Wilson & McLean 1989).

According to behavioral components, not type of disability, we will have two different approaches for operative techniques.

1.  *Uncooperative behavior*—restorative treatment has to rely on behavior management/guidance techniques and atraumatic restorative treatment (ART). This is removal of just the carious lesion with hand instruments. After the removal, and without extending the area, it is filled with glass ionomer cement.

2. *Cooperative behavior*—this is a noninvasive technique, mechanically removing all the affected areas of enamel and dentin, leaving a clear and clean preparation border, using a small round or pear-shaped bur. Glass ionomer can be placed directly in the preparation serving three physic-mechanical means: (a) as a *cavity protective baseline*, (b) as the *filling itself*, and (c) as a *fluoride-releasing factor* in the oral cavity that appears to assist in remineralization of the affected dentin under a carious lesion.

Make sure you develop a clean margin around the lesion to ensure a complete seal through adhesion. Moisture control is still essential but the shorter time for placement means that there is less time for contamination (Gryst & Mount 1999). Where occlusal load is expected to be too heavy to be sustained by glass ionomer alone, an alternative is the combination of a resin composite/glass ionomer using the laminating technique (Mount 1989).

*Stainless steel crowns* are still considered by some practitioners to be the definite restoration for primary and permanent molars. These are used in patients without DDDs, as a rule, but adapting these crowns for optimal gingival fit and minimal inflammation in primary or permanent molars is difficult. So, again, every patient will require a different approach based on gingival health. Crowns should be cemented with glass ionomer or polycarboxilate cement. Ng et al. (2001) found a significantly higher stainless steel crown failure rate in young patients with DDDs.

A *removable partial denture* (RPD) is easier to repair and replace than a cast restoration, and there is often an aesthetic advantage for patients with cerebral palsy and intellectual disability. We have to take into consideration that an RPD is more fragile and more susceptible to trauma from seizures. There should be a concern for aspiration of fragments after traumatic injuries. The appliance could be modified with acrylic teeth and a wire mesh reinforced acrylic. A major concern with some levels of disability is oral hygiene and the care of the appliance. Griess et al. (1998) reported acceptable success rates of comprehensive prosthetic procedures for disabled patients. On the other hand, Durham et al. (2006) reported that behavior during the restorative process, prosthetic complications from post placement, and patient's oral hygiene should influence patient selection and prosthetic design.

*Endodontic* treatments depend again on the behavior aspects of the patient. If no radiograph is possible, we know that endodontic therapy can be accomplished, but it reduces considerably the chance of success. It may be preferable to extract the tooth. Sometimes, when a true endodontic therapy cannot be performed, a pulpotomy may be performed whenever we believe there is a chance for pulp survival. It is believed that this is a compromise and a less ideal endodontic therapy than other alternatives to extraction, especially in a patient for whom tooth replacement is not an important expectation.

*Orthodontic therapy* can be accomplished on some patients with DDDs who are able to cooperate but may not be considered for patients who are not successful with behavior management/guidance techniques. Again, patient cooperation will be the key factor in determining success. There are some exceptions that tolerate the treatment and, of course, benefit from the treatment.

*Exodontia* and/or *oral surgery* of teeth with poor or bad prognosis is less indicated when there is no possibility for a prostheses replacement. Patients with DDDs often experience the presence of impacted teeth and the clinician is faced with a difficult decision: to monitor or extract. If the decision is to monitor, the clinician has to understand that a comprehensive oral hygiene plan must be established in order to decrease plaque formation.

## SUMMARY

People with DDDs present with many challenges that are unique to their condition. Providing oral health services to patients with disabilities requires an adjustment of our everyday skills. The dental professional must have a clear knowledge of the condition and personalize individual treatment plans according to each patient's needs. This chapter has described strategies of care that lead to successful restorative appointments for patients with DDDs. In addition, material selection will ultimately depend on the patient's specific condition and behavior status.

## REFERENCES

Abbud R, Ferreira LA, Campos AG, et al. (2002). Atendimiento clínico de emergencia: un etudo do servicios oferecidos en dez anos (Portuguese). *Revista da Associacao Paulista de Cirurgioes Dentistas* 56(4):271–275.

American Dental Association. (2000). *Guidelines for the use of conscious sedation, deep sedation and general anesthesia for dentists.* Chicago: American Dental Association.

———. (2008). Americans with Disabilities Act 2008, Public Law 110-325. Accessed from www.ada.gov/pubs/adastatute08.htm.

Baker R. (1990). Development of a questionnaire to access patient's satisfaction with consultations in general practices. *British Journal of General Practice* 40:487–490.

Bates MN, Fawcett J, Garrett N, et al. (2004). Health effects of dental amalgam exposure: A retrospective cohort study. *International Journal of Epidemiology* 33(4):894–902.

Beck JD, Hunt RJ. (1985). Oral health status in the United States: Problems of special patients. *Journal of Dental Education* 49:407–425.

Bellinger DC, Daniel D, Trachtenberg F, et al. (2007a). Dental amalgam restorations and children's neuropsychological function: The New England Children's Amalgam Trial. *Environmental Health Perspectives* 115(3):440–446.

Bellinger DC, Trachtenberg F, Daniel D, et al. (2007b). A dose-effect analysis of children's exposure to dental amalgam and neuropsychological function: The New England Children's Amalgam Trial. *Journal of the American Dental Association* 138(9)1210–1216.

Bellinger DC, Trachtenberg F, Zhang A, et al. (2008). Dental amalgam and psychosocial status: The New England Children's Amalgam Trial. *Journal of Dental Research* 87(5):470–474.

Da Costa SL, Malm O, Dorea JG. (2005). Breast milk mercury concentrations and amalgam surface in mothers from Brasilia, Brazil. *Biological Trace Element Research* 106(2):145–151.

Daniels JL, Rowland AS, Longnecker MP, et al. (2007). Maternal dental history: Child's birth outcomes and early cognitive development. ALSPAC Study Team. *Paediatric and Perinatal Epidemiology* 21(5):448–457.

Davidson PW, Myers GJ, Weiss B. (2004). Mercury and child development outcomes. *Pediatrics* 113:1023–1029.

Drasch G, Schupp I, Hofl H, et al. (1994). Mercury burden of human fetal and infant tissues. *European Journal of Pediatrics* 153:607–610.

Durham TM, King T, Salinas T, et al. (2006). Dental implants in edentulous adults with cognitive disabilities: Report of the pilot project. *Special Care in Dentistry* 26(1):40–46.

Ellis RK, Donly KJ, Wild TW. (1992). Indirect composite resin crowns as an esthetic approach to treating ectodermal dysplasia: A case report. *Quintessence International* 23(11):727–729.

Feldman CA, Giringer M, Sanders M, et al. (1997). Special Olympics, Special Smiles: Assessing the feasibility of epidemiologic data collection. *Journal of the American Dental Association* 128:1687–1696.

Forsten L. (1994). Fluoride release of glass ionomers. In P. Hunt (Ed.), *Glass Ionomers: The Next Generation* (pp. 241–244). Philadelphia: International Symposia in Dentistry.

Garcia–Godoy FM. (2009). *Handbook of Prenatal and Postnatal Preventive Dentistry* (Spanish). Santo Domingo: AIBOFA, Iberoamerican Graduate Dental School Publications, INCE University, pp. 142–157.

———. (2010a). Communication with the child: Non-pharmacological behaviour management. In F.M. Garcia–Godoy & C. Garcia–Godoy, *Handbook of Clinical Pediatric Dentistry* (in Spanish) (pp. 101–114). Santo Domingo: AIBOFA.

———. (2010b). The big C: Multifactorial response of tooth and biofilm to all determinants of the infection. In F.M. Garcia-Godoy, F. Garcia-Godoy F, & C. Garcia-Godoy, *Manual de Odontologia Preventiva Prenatal y Postnatal* (in Spanish) (p. 135). Santo Domingo: AIBOFA.

Geier DA, Kern JK, Geier MR. (2009). A prospective study of prenatal mercury exposure from maternal dental amalgams and autism severity. *Acta Neurobiologiae Experimentalis* 69(2):189–197.

Girdler NM, Hill CM. (1988). Spectrum of patient management. In *Sedation in Dentistry* (p. 3). Oxford: Butterworth-Heinemann.

Grandjean P, White RF, Nielsen A, et al. (1999). Methylmercury neurotoxicity in Amazonian children downstream from gold mining. *Environmental Health Perspectives* 107:587–591.

Griess M, Reilmann B, Chanavaz M. (1998). The multi-modal prosthetic treatment of mentally handicapped patients—necessity and challenge. *European Journal of Prosthodontics and Restorative Dentistry* 6(3):115–120.

Gryst MEI, Mount GJ. (1999). The use of glass ionomer in special needs patients. *Australian Dental Journal* 44(4):268–274.

Hall JA, Roter DL, Katz NR. (1987). Task versus socio-emotional behaviors in physicians. *Medical Care* 25(5):399–412.

Harada Y. (1968). Congenital (or fetal) Minamata Disease. In *Minamata Disease* (pp. 93–118). Kumamoto, Japan: Kumamoto University.

Havio ML. (1995). Oral health care of the mentally retarded and other persons with disabilities in the Nordic countries: Present situation and plans for the future. *Special Care in Dentistry* 15:16–19.

Hujoel PP, Lydon-Rochelle M, Bollen AM, et al. (2005). Mercury exposure from dental fillings placement during pregnancy and low birth weight risk. *American Journal of Epidemiology* 161(8):734–740.

Kingsman A, Albers JW, Arezzo JC, et al. (2005). Amalgam exposure and neurologic function. *Neurotoxicology* 26(2):241–255.

Kjellstrom T, Kennedy P, Wallis S, et al. (1989). *Physical and mental development of children with prenatal exposure to mercury from fish*. Stage II: Interviews and psychological tests at age 6. Solna, Sweden: National Swedish Environmental Protection Board. (Report 3642).

Lauterbach M, Martins IP, Castro–Caldas A, Bernardo M, Luis H, Amaral H, Leitao J, Martin MD, Townes B, Rosenbaum G, Woods JS, Derouen T. (2008). Neurological outcomes in children with and without amalgam–related mercury exposure: Seven years of longitudinal observations in a randomized trail. *Journal of the American dental Association* 139: 138–145.

Lester GW, Smith SG. (1993). Listening and talking to patients: A remedy for malpractice. *Western Journal of Medicine* 158(3):268–272.

Lindbohm ML, Ylöstalo P, Sallmen M, et al. (2007). Occupational exposure in dentistry and miscarriage. *Occupational and Environmental Medicine* 64(2):127–133.

Luglie PF, Campus G, Chessa G, et al. (2005). Effect of amalgam fillings on the mercury concentration in human amniotic fluid. *Archives of Gynecology and Obstetrics* 271(2):138–142.

Mani SP, Cleaton-Jones PE, Lownie JF. (1997). Demographic profile of patients who went for emergency treatment at WIT's Dental School. *Journal of the Dental Assocation of South Africa* 52(2):69–72.

Marsh D, Turner M, Santos J, et al. (1995). Fetal methyl mercury study in a Peruvian fish-eating population. *Neurotoxicology* 16:717–726.

Mckeown-Eyssen G, Reudy J, Neims A. (1983). Methylmercury exposures in Northern Quebec II: Neurologic findings in children. *American Journal of Epidemiology* 118:470–479.

Mount GJ. (1989). Clinical requirements for a successful "sandwich" dentin to glass ionomer cement to composite resin. *Australian Dental Journal* 34:159–165.

National Association of the Deaf. (1990). Americans with Disabilities Act. Accessed from http://www.nad.org/issues/civil-rights/ADA.

Ng MW, Tate AR, Needleman NL, et al. (2001). The influence of medical history on restorative procedures failure rates following dental rehabilitation. *Pediatric Dentistry* 23:487–490.

Palkovicova L, Ursinyova M, Masanova V, et al. (2008). Maternal amalgam dental fillings as the source of mercury exposure in developing fetus and newborns. *Journal of Exposure Science and Environmental Epidemiology* 18(3):326–331.

Pyles DAM, Muniz K, Cade A, Silva R. (1997). A behavioral diagnostic paradigm for integrating behavior-analytical and psychopharmacological intervention in people with a dual diagnosis. *Research in Developmental Disabilities* 18(3):185–214.

Ramirez GB, Cruz CV, Pagulayan O, et al. (2000). The Tagum Study I: Analysis and clinical correlates of mercury in maternal and cord blood, breast milk, meconium, and infant's hair. *Pediatrics* 116:774–781.

Raposa K. (2009). Behavioral management for patients with intellectual and developmental disorders. *Dental Clinics of North America* 53(2):359–373, xi.

Smith DC, Williams DF. (1982). *Biocompatibility of dental materials*. Boca Raton, FL: CRC Press.

U.S. Department of Health and Human Services. (2009). National Institutes of Health. National Institute of Dental and Craniofacial research. Practical oral care for people with development disabilities: Health challenges and strategies for care. Continuing Education NIH 09-5196.

U.S. Department of Health and Human Services. (2005–2006). *The National Survey of Children with Special Health Care Needs. Chartbook*. Rockville, MD: Department of Health and Human Services, p. 35.

Waldman HB. (2005). Preparing dental graduates to provide care to individuals with special needs. *Journal of Dental Education* 69(2):249–254.

Waldman HB, Perlman SP. (2010). Disability and rehabilitation: Do we ever think about needed dental care? A case study: The USA. *Disability and Rehabilitation* 32(11):947–951.

Waldman HB, Perlman SP, Swerdlof M. (2000). Use of pediatric dental services in the 1990: Some continuing difficulties. *Journal of Dentistry for Children* 67:59–63.

Waldman HB, Rader R, Perlman SP. (2009). Health related issues for individuals with special health care needs. *Dental Clinics of North America* 53:183–193.

Wilson GJ, McLean JW. (1989). *Glass-Ionomer Cement*. London: Quintessence.

Wilson KI. (1992). Treatment accessibility for physically and mentally handicapped people—a review of the literature. *Community Dental Health* 9: 187–192.

Ye X, Quian H, Xu P, et al. (2009). Nephrotoxicity and mercury exposure among children with and without dental amalgam fillings. *International Journal of Hygiene and Environmental Health* 212(4):378–386.

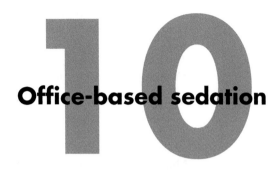

# Office-based sedation

Matthew Cooke, DDS, MD, MPH

The goal of this chapter is to aid the dentist and dental hygienist in managing pain and anxiety and modifying behavior to safely complete dental procedures in patients with developmental disorders. Developmental and chronologic age both affect a patient's ability to control his or her behavior for a dental procedure (AAPD 2007–2008; Maxwell & Yaster 1996). Young patients and severely developmentally disabled patients may require deeper levels of sedation to gain control of their behavior (Maxwell & Yaster 1996). Therefore, the dentist should consider the need for deep sedation. However, for more cooperative patients, traditional behavior management/ guidance such as distraction, tell-show-do, guided imagery, topical anesthesia, and hypnosis may reduce the need for or depth of pharmacologic sedation (AAPD 2007–2008; Kennedy & Luchman 1999; Newton et al. 2003).

## DEFINITIONS

Many definitions of sedation for dentistry have been used over the years. The most recent documents defining sedation and anesthesia are from the House of Delegates Meeting of the American Dental Association (ADA) in 2007 (ADA 2007a, 2007b). Clinical standards for sedation in dentistry parallel the guidelines established by the American Society of Anesthesiologists (ASA 2002). The American Academy of Pediatric Dentistry (AAPD) and the

*Treating the Dental Patient with a Developmental Disorder*, First Edition.
Edited by Karen A. Raposa and Steven P. Perlman.
© 2012 John Wiley & Sons, Inc. Published 2012 by John Wiley & Sons, Inc.

American Academy of Pediatrics (AAP) also maintain guidelines for sedation of the pediatric patient, defined as any patient under the age of 21 (AAPD 2007–2008).

The following definitions for levels of sedation are excerpted from the ADA, AAPD, and AAP guidelines (AAPD 2007–2008; ADA 2007a, 2007b):

**Minimal sedation** (old terminology "anxiolysis"): a drug-induced state during which patients respond normally to verbal commands. Although cognitive function and coordination may be impaired, ventilatory and cardiovascular functions are unaffected.

**Moderate sedation** (old terminology "conscious sedation" or "sedation/ analgesia"): a drug-induced depression of consciousness during which patients respond purposefully to verbal commands (e.g., "open your eyes" either alone or accompanied by light tactile stimulation—a light tap on the shoulder or face, not a sternal rub). For older patients, this level of sedation implies an interactive state; for younger patients, age-appropriate behaviors (e.g., crying) occur and are expected.

Note: "In accord with this particular definition, the drug(s) and/or techniques used should carry a margin of safety wide enough to render loss of consciousness unlikely. Repeated dosing of an agent before the effects of previous dosing can be fully appreciated may result in a greater alteration of the state of consciousness than is the intent of the dentist. Further, patients whose only response is reflex withdrawal from repeated painful stimuli would not be considered to be in a state of moderate sedation" (Malamed 2010).

**Deep sedation** (deep sedation/analgesia): a drug-induced depression of consciousness during which patients cannot be easily aroused but respond purposefully after repeated verbal or painful stimulation. The ability to independently maintain ventilatory function may be impaired. Patients may require assistance in maintaining a patent airway, and spontaneous ventilation may be inadequate. Cardiovascular function is usually maintained. A state of deep sedation may be accompanied by partial or complete loss of protective reflexes.

**General anesthesia**: a drug-induced loss of consciousness during which patients are not arousable, even by painful stimulation. The ability to independently maintain ventilatory function is often impaired. Patients often require assistance in maintaining a patent airway, and positive pressure ventilation may be required because of depressed spontaneous ventilation or drug-induced depression of neuromuscular function. Cardiovascular function may be impaired.

## SPECTRUM OF ANESTHESIA AND SEDATION

In 1937, Arthur Guedel, MD, introduced the concept of anesthetic signs and stages. His early work was based on the use of di-ethyl ether for general

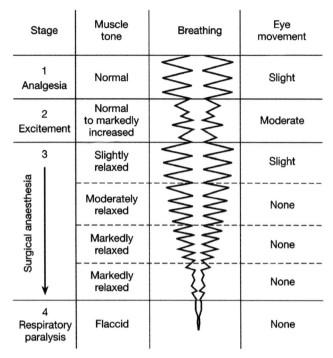

| Stage | Muscle tone | Breathing | Eye movement |
|---|---|---|---|
| 1<br>Analgesia | Normal | | Slight |
| 2<br>Excitement | Normal to markedly increased | | Moderate |
| 3 | Slightly relaxed | | Slight |
| | Moderately relaxed | | None |
| | Markedly relaxed | | None |
| | Markedly relaxed | | None |
| 4<br>Respiratory paralysis | Flaccid | | None |

**Figure 10.1**   Guedel's early work.

anesthesia. He showed that as patients were administered increasing quantities of ether they moved through four distinct stages. The stages represent a continuum or spectrum progressing from no sedation to general anesthesia (Douglas 1958).

Figure 10.1 illustrates Guedel's early work graphically. (Harrison-Calmes 2002). In stage 1, the analgesia phase, consciousness is not lost. Between stages 2 and 3, consciousness is lost. Dentists who have not been trained in the use of deep sedation and general anesthesia need to limit their practice to stage 1, the analgesia phase.

Although Guedel's work is still tenable, it has been revised and adapted to include new drugs and techniques. This is particularly true as it relates to ambulatory sedation and anesthesia for dental procedures. The dentist must understand that as drugs are given they produce an outcome along a *"spectrum of pain and anxiety control"* (Malamed 2010). Different drugs administered via different routes will produce various levels of sedation or anesthesia.

Figure 10.2 shows the spectrum. At the left there is no sedation or anesthesia. Moving right, there are levels of conscious sedation up to the vertical bar. The bar represents loss of consciousness. To the right of the bar is deep sedation/general anesthesia. It is paramount that the dentist understands where he or she is on the spectrum and where he or she wants to be.

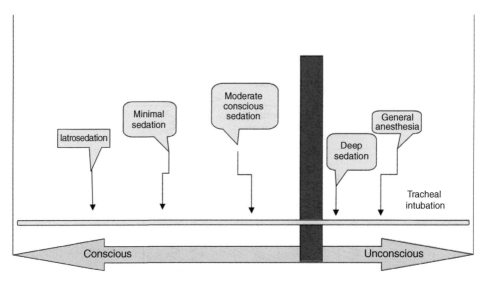

**Figure 10.2**   Sedation spectrum.

## Rescue

The concept of "rescue" is essential to safe sedation. Recognizing that levels of sedation and anesthesia are along a continuum, it is paramount that the provider be able to rescue a patient from unintended entry to a more profound level of CNS depression (AAPD 2007–2008; Malamed 2010; Cote et al. 2000; Hoffman et al. 2002; AHA 2002). The ASA in their guidelines include and stress the concept of rescue during the administration of sedation by "non-anesthesiologists" in an effort to reduce morbidity and mortality.

> Because sedation is a continuum, it is not always possible to predict how an individual patient will respond. Hence, practitioners intending to produce a given level of sedation should be able to rescue patients whose level of sedation becomes deeper than initially intended. Individuals administering Moderate Sedation should be able to rescue patients who enter a state of deep sedation, while those administering deep sedation should be able to rescue patients who enter a state of general anesthesia (ASA 2002).

Sedation can also be accomplished without the use of drugs. It is known as iatrosedation. Techniques include acupressure, acupuncture, biofeedback, electronic dental anesthesia, and hypnosis (Malamed 2010). Iatrosedation may provide an alternative to traditional sedation and/or general anesthesia for patients with developmental disorders. However, for purposes of this chapter, we will focus on the use of pharmacotherapy to obtain a desired outcome.

Communication is the key to successful sedation. The dentist and dental hygienist cannot ignore the power of good communication with the patient. Knowing the patient's developmental and chronological age will help the provider meet the patient at his or her level. There is no substitute for good verbal and nonverbal communication that is developmentally age appropriate. It has been shown that good communication has the potential to remove a patient's fear and anxiety and allow treatment to proceed in a "normal" fashion (Malamed 2010). More often, however, good communication facilitates the acceptance of pharmacosedation with a successful outcome.

# PHYSICAL STATUS CLASSIFICATION

Dental treatment can have profound effects on both the physical and psychological "well-being" of patients with developmental disorders. It is important that prior to any dental treatment a complete physical and psychological assessment be done. This information is necessary to provide high-quality care and prevent serious complications.

Physical and psychological assessments allow the dentist to determine if a patient will tolerate a procedure and/or determine if an alternative modality is needed. Medical and psychological histories should guide the dentist in choosing a treatment modality. Physical evaluation should include a medical history questionnaire, a physical examination, and a discussion with the patient, parent, and/or caregiver. With information collected, the dentist can establish a physical status classification and determine risk factors. Medical consults can be obtained as needed and the appropriate treatment planned, which may include pharmacosedation (Malamed 2010).

In 1962, the ASA adopted a classification system for estimating medical risk for a patient receiving general anesthesia for a surgical procedure. It is what is now referred to as the ASA Physical Status (PS) Classification System (ASA 1963). The system has remained virtually unchanged and has since been adopted for evaluation of medical risk associated with all surgical procedures regardless of anesthetic technique (Fleisher 2005; Lagasse 2002).

The ASA Physical Status Classification System (ASA 1963):

**ASA PS 1**: a healthy patient (no physiologic, physical, or psychological abnormalities).

**ASA PS 2**: a patient with mild systemic disease without limitation of daily activities (i.e., controlled asthma; controlled hypertension).

**ASA PS 3**: a patient with severe systemic disease that limits activity but is not incapacitating (i.e., uncontrolled hypertension; uncontrolled diabetes).

**ASA PS 4**: a patient with incapacitating systemic disease that is a constant threat to life.

**ASA PS 5**: a moribund patient not expected to survive 24 hours without the operation.

**ASA PS 6**: a brain-dead patient whose organs are being removed for donor purposes.

If the procedure to be performed is an emergency an "E" is added to the above classification system (e.g., ASA PS 2E). In outpatient medical and dental settings ASA PS 5 and ASA PS 6 have been eliminated (ASA 1963).

Patients who are ASA PS 1 and 2 are generally considered appropriate candidates for minimal, moderate, or deep sedation in the dental office (AAPD 2007–2008). Most mild developmental disorders are ASA PS 2 patients. Individuals in the ASA PS classes 3 and 4 require individual consideration, particularly for moderate and deep sedation (AAPD 2007–2008; Malviya et al. 1997). Dentists are encouraged to consult with appropriate subspecialties when necessary for patients at increased risk. Remember, the ultimate responsibility and liability rest with the dentist who decides to treat or not treat.

# SEDATION

The sedation of patients with developmental disorders needing oral health care represents a unique clinical challenge. Consideration must be given to such factors as the patient's age and corresponding levels of cognitive and coping skills. Because of patient extremes in responsiveness and acceptability of treatment modalities, the intended goals and outcomes of sedation will vary depending on a host of factors. These guidelines should aid clinicians in achieving the benefits of sedation while minimizing associated risks and adverse outcomes for the patient.

The ideal sedation should:

1. Be safe.
2. Be easy to administer.
3. Have rapid and reliable onset.
4. Alleviate pain and anxiety.
5. Have minimal undesirable side effects.
6. Be reversible.

Once the decision has been made to use pharmacosedation, the dentist must consider what drugs to use and how to administer the drug. Choosing a method for delivery to a patient with a developmental disorder will vary depending on desired level of sedation and the patient's willingness to cooperate. Cooperative patients with developmental disorders who require less sedation often receive sedative agents via the oral route, whereas uncooperative patients with limited cognitive skills often require induction via the intra-muscular route followed by an IV to administer additional agents.

Drugs may be administered to the patient with a developmental disorder via the following routes:

1. Oral/rectal.
2. Topical.
3. Intranasal.
4. Inhalational.
5. Sublingual/transmucosal.
6. Subcutaneous.
7. Intramuscular (IM).
8. Intravenous (IV).
9. Intraarterial (IA).
10. Intrathecal (in spinal fluid).
11. Transdermal (through epidermis).

Oral and rectal sedation are termed enteral sedation. The drug is administered directly into the gastrointestinal tract (GI) with systemic absorbtion occuring across the entire membrane. This is different from other routes in which drug absorption occurs directly into the systemic circulation, known as parenteral sedation.

The oral route is the most popular route used for sedation in dentistry. It has several advantages over the parenteral routes, which include acceptance by patients, low cost, ease of administration, decreased incidence of adverse reaction, and no equipment needed for delivery (Malamed 2010). However, oral sedation does have some significant disadvantages, such as reliance on patient compliance, a prolonged latent period, erratic and incomplete absorption from the GI tract, inability to titrate, inability to lighten or deepen sedation as needed, and a prolonged duration of action. With oral sedation, adding more medicine after the initial dose is usually not recommended.

The rectal route is similar to the oral route in its advantages and disadvantages. It is primarily used in diaper-age patients and patients who are either unwilling or unable to take drugs by mouth (Malamed 2010; Flaitz 1986; Jensen & Matsson 2001). The rectal route bypasses a portion of the GI tract (stomach), therefore a quicker and more profound sedation may be noticed. As with oral sedation, it is not recommended to add additional medicine after the initial dose.

Topical administration of a drug works well for nonkeratinized skin. Therefore, topical anesthetics are highly effective at relieving pain associated with intraoral injections of local anesthesia (Carr & Horton 2001). Topical applications of drugs in dentistry are usually limited to local anesthetics. With topical anesthetics there is more allergic potential (localized, not systemic) because of their benzocaine-based formulation.

Intranasal administration has become increasingly popular in pediatrics. It is easily administered to resistant, uncooperative, or precooperative patients (Malamed 2010; Fukota et al. 1993; Fuks et al. 1994; Lam et al. 2005). Although there is brief discomfort with administration, absorption is directly into the systemic circulation, making the drug rapidly bioavailable. There is reduced time to onset and total time spent in the office, when compared with oral sedation. Midazolam, a water-soluble benzodiazepine, is the most commonly used drug via the intra-nasal route (Malamed 2010; Fukota et al. 1993; Fuks et al. 1994; Lam et al. 2005; Walbergh et al. 1991). The mucosal atomization device (MAD) is the preferred method for nasal administration.

Inhalation drug administration is when gaseous agents pass from the nose or mouth to the trachea and lungs into the cardiovascular system. There are a variety of agents available for inhalational sedation and anesthesia. In dentistry, nitrous oxide/oxygen sedation is the main drug used for inhalation sedation (Malamed 2010; Jastak & Donaldson 1991). It is easily titrated to effect, with minimal side effects or complications. Disadvantages of nitrous oxide are that it is not a potent anesthetic, so there may be failure. Also, a delivery system is required with a fail-safe and scavenging system. The equipment must be calibrated annually and there needs to be adequate office ventilation to prevent chronic exposure to personnel administering the sedation.

Sublingual drugs are administered under or beneath the tongue (hypoglossal). Transmucosal drugs are delivered through mucous membranes. With sublingual and transmucosal administration, the drug enters directly into the systemic circulation, bypassing the enterohepatic system. Avoidance of the hepatic first-pass effect makes the drug rapidly bioavailable. Nitroglycerin, for relief of anginal pain, is an example of a drug commonly given via the sublingual and transmucosal route. In dentistry, benzodiazepines and opiates for sedation and pain control may be delivered via the sublingual or oral transmucosal route (Malamed 2010; Hosaka et al. 2009). This route of delivery may have limited application for the noncooperative patient, such as one with a moderate to severe developmental disorder.

Subcutaneous injection is where the drug is administered beneath the skin into the subcutaneous tissue. The rate of absorption into the CVS is directly proportional to the vasculature in the area of injection. The slow rate of absorption may limit the usefulness in dentistry.

The intra-muscular route is a parenteral technique in which the drug is injected directly into the muscle. Advantages include rapid onset and rapid onset of maximal clinical effect. Disadvantages are prolonged deep sedation, possible injury to tissues at injection site, and overdose. This route of administration is often not predictable and does not allow for titration to effect. Ketamine, a dissociative anesthetic, is the most commonly used drug via the intramuscular route and is often used for sedation and induction of the uncooperative patient with a developmental disorder (Sinner & Graf 2008). Skilled and experienced anesthesia providers familiar with anatomy may inject ketamine through the clothing of uncooperative patients with developmental disorders.

The intravenous route of drug administration represents the most effective method of predictable adequate sedation for most patients (Malamed 2010). Advantages to this route include rapid onset with short duration of latent period, and a shortened recovery. Disadvantages include complications at venipuncture site and risk for overdose. IVs may often be difficult to obtain on patients with developmental disorders. Many drugs given via IV do not have reversals; therefore the dentist must be prepared to manage deeper sedation and other complications such as allergic reactions, which may not be seen with other less effective modes of delivery (Malamed 2010).

A variety of drugs are available for sedation of the patient with a developmental disorder. These primarily include nitrous oxide/oxygen inhalation sedation, benzodiazepines, sedative hypnotics, and opioids. Table 10.1 lists available drugs for sedation.

**Table 10.1** Commonly Used Drugs for Sedation of the Patient with a Developmental Disorder

| | |
|---|---|
| Inhalation Agents | Barbiturates |
|   Nitrous Oxide/Oxygen Sedation |   Methohexital |
| Benzodiazepines |   Sodium Thiopental |
|   Diazepam | Hypnotics |
|   Midazolam |   Chloral Hydrate |
|   Lorazepam | Alpha Agonists |
|   Triazolam |   Clonidine |
| Opioid Agonists |   Dexmedetomidine |
|   Fentanyl | Antihistamines |
|   Morphine |   Hydroxyzine |
|   Meperidine |   Diphenhydramine |
|   Alfentanil, Sufentanil and Remifentanil* |   Promethazine |
| Dissociative Anesthetics | Anticholinergics |
|   Ketamine* |   Atropine |
| Propofol* |   Scopolamine |
| |   Glycopyrrolate |

*Not recommended for use in IV moderate sedation without anesthesia training.

The goal for choosing a sedation regimen for patients with developmental disorders can best be achieved by selecting the lowest dose of drug with the highest therapeutic index for the planned procedure. The regimen needs to account for any physical, developmental, mental, sensory, behavioral, cognitive, or emotional impairment that limits the patient's ability to cooperate. Selection of the fewest number of drugs paired with the goal of the procedure is essential for safe practice (Mace et al. 2004; Deshpande & Tobias 1996; Alcaino 2000; Malviya et al. 2001; Yaster et al. 1997; Cravero & Blike 2004; Krauss & Green 2006). This means if a painful procedure is planned, an opiate may be the drug of choice. If the procedure is more diagnostic, a sedative may be more appropriate. Combinations of different classes are often used. However, when three-plus agents are used together the potential for an adverse outcome increases (ASA 2002; Mitchell et al. 1982). The dentist also must be prepared for paradoxical reactions, the opposite of the desired outcome, in patients with developmental disorders.

# DRUGS AVAILABLE FOR SEDATION OF PATIENTS WITH DEVELOPMENTAL DISORDERS

## Nitrous oxide/oxygen sedation

Short-term exposure to nitrous oxide includes sedation, euphoria, giddiness, elation, and a general sense of well-being. Nitrous oxide is the least potent of the inhalation anesthetics, but in dentistry it is the most frequently used (Malamed 2010). The MAC (minimum alveolar concentration of an agent that prevents movement in 50% of patients to a surgical incision) for nitrous oxide is 105%. It is difficult to reach this level unless it is administered under hyperbaric conditions (Malamed 2010). However, Guadel's stage 2, delirium, can be reached if nitrous oxide is not properly administered (Douglas 1958; Harrison-Calmes 2002). Nitrous oxide may be administered alone or in combination with other agents.

Nitrous oxide (Figures 10.3a through 10.3c) is a safe, affordable option for conscious sedation of many patients with developmental disorders. There are relatively few absolute contraindications to nitrous oxide as long as the percentage of oxygen administered is not allowed to go below 21% that of ambient air, which is unlikely because of built in fail-safe mechanisms (Clark & Brunick 2008). However, there are a few relative complications, such as patients with compulsive personalities, claustrophobia, personality disorders, upper respiratory tract infections (URIs), chronic obstructive pulmonary disease (COPD), pregnancy, and children with severe behavioral issues (Malamed 2010).

### Fundamental principles for appropriate administration of nitrous oxide/oxygen sedation ($N_2O/O_2$)

- Be enthusiastic and confident that the experience will be positive.
- Be knowledgeable about the limits of this mild sedative.
- Recognize that patients in your care represent the best opportunity you have to express genuine care and concern.

(a)                              (b)                              (c)

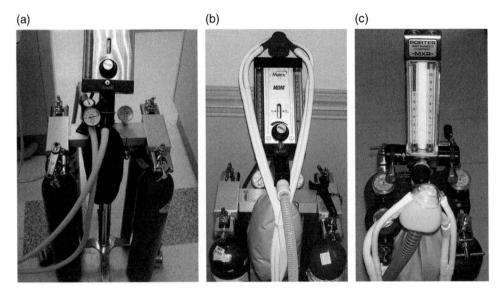

**Figure 10.3a–10.3c**    Nitrous oxide.

- Informed consent must be obtained for each patient before $N_2O/O_2$ administration.
- Practice titration by adjusting the concentration to stress of the procedure.
- Begin and end with 100% oxygen.
- The patient should not be left alone.
- Accurately document all procedures, nitrous oxide/oxygen dose, reactions, complications, and so forth, in patient's record.
- Place patient in comfortable position before administration.
- Inform the patient to ask for assistance at any time in the procedure if needed.
- If nitrous oxide is to be used at the next appointment, recommend that the patient not have a large meal prior to the appointment.

Titrate to the level of sedation that is determined by patient comfort and relaxation. There is no fixed percentage of $N_2O/O_2$ for sedation for a given experience or patient. There is also no preset LPM (liters per minute) of $N_2O/O_2$. The percentage of $N_2O/O_2$ given to a patient or experience will not reflect the amount necessary for any other experience. The goal is to keep the patient relaxed and comfortable. (Clark & Brunick 1999, 2008)

Generally emergence from nitrous oxide is a mirror image of induction. The mirror image includes the patient returning to his or her original emotional state, as well as recovering from the pharmacological effects. Terminate nitrous oxide flow; continue delivering 100% oxygen during the final minutes of the procedure. This begins the postoperative oxygenation phase of 3–5 minutes, at which point the patient should be completely recovered (Jastak & Orendruff 1975).

Nitrous oxide/oxygen sedation may be used to augment an oral sedation. This can add a degree of safety because the patient is getting a minimum of 30% oxygen, which is greater than the 21% of room air. Some state regulations do not allow polypharmacy, so augmentation may not be an option.

## Benzodiazepines

The benzodiazepines have become the most popular and widely used sedatives in dentistry for patients with developmental disorders. Benzodiazepines bind the GABA-A receptor and inhibit central nervous system function, mainly in the thalamus and limbic systems, the area of the brain responsible for emotion and behavior (Giovannitti & Moore 2011). Benzodiazepines are reversible with flumazenil and have a wide safety margin (therapeutic dose to toxic dose), making them desirable for sedation in dentistry. Tables 10.2 and 10.3 show available benzodiazepines used in anxiolysis and sedation with dosages for the average adult sized patient.

Midazolam (Dormicum or Versed), a short-acting water-soluble benzodiazepine, is perhaps the most popular agent. It is the mainstay of pediatric sedation and premedicatation for patients with developmental disorders (Parnis et al. 1992; Feld et al. 1990). It causes sedation with antegrade amnesia; it has a relatively short half-life and can be reversed (Conner et al. 1978; Hennesy et al. 1991; Longmire & Seger 1993).

### *Midazolam and routes of administration*

1. *IM*—not well accepted and should be reserved for difficult patients. Dose: 0.1–0.2 mg/kg, which peaks in 15 minutes.
2. *IV*—venous access required. Smaller therapeutic index. Caution when used with opioids for premedication due to its blunting of hypoxic ventilatory drive.
3. *Oral*—most popular but difficult to mask bitter taste. Optimal separation from parents in 30–45 minutes. Dose: 0.5 mg/kg up to total of 15 mg max.
4. *Rectal*—most often used in diaper-age patients. Maximum plasma level is in 19–29 minutes. Disadvantage is variation in absorption and sometimes causes defecation. Dose: 0.4–1.0 mg/kg.
5. *Nasal*—acidic solution that burns. May be poor absorption in cases of URI with increased nasal secretions. Sedation occurs in 7–10 minutes. Dose: 0.2–0.3 mg/kg.
6. *Oral transmucosal*—sublingual. Very effective but not good in young or noncompliant children because of bitter taste. Dose: 0.1–0.2 mg/kg.

**Table 10.2**  Benzodiazepines for oral use (Malamed 2010).

| Generic name | Brand | Class* | Availability (mg) | Dose (mg) |
|---|---|---|---|---|
| Alprazolam | Xanax | AA | 0.25,0.5,1 | 0.25–0.5 |
| Chlordiazepide | Librium | AA | 5,10,25 | 10 |
| Clonazepam | Klonopin | AC | 0.5,1,2 | |
| Diazepam | Valium | AA | 2,5,10 | 10 |
| Flunitrazepam | Rohypnol | SH | 2 | 0.25–2 |
| Flurazepam | Dalmane | SH | 15,30 | 30 |
| Halazepam | Paxipam | AA | 20,40 | 20–40 |
| Lorazepam | Ativan | SH, AA | 0.5,1,2 | 2–4 |
| Medazepam | Nobrium | AA | 5,10 | 5–10 |
| Midazolam | Dormicum | SH | 15 | 15–30 |
| Oxazepam | Serax | AA | 10,15,30 | 15–30 |
| Prazepam | Centrax | AA | 5,10 | 10–20 |
| Temazepam | Restoril | SH | 15,30 | 30 |
| Triazolam | Halcion | SH | 0.25,0.5 | 0.25–0.5 |

*AA = anti-anxiety; AC = anti-convulsant; SH = sedative-hypnotic.

**Table 10.3**  Benzodiazepines for intravenous moderate sedation.

| Generic Name | Brand | Concentration (mg/ml) | Average dose (mg) |
|---|---|---|---|
| Diazepam | Valium | 5 | 10–12 |
| Lorazepam | Ativan | 2 | 2–4 |
| Midazolam | Versed | 1 | 2.5–7.5 |

Benzodiazepines frequently induce sedation; however, paradoxical reactions have been observed (Carissa et al. 2004). These reactions are described as increased talkativeness, emotional release, excitement, and excessive movement. Paradoxical reactions are more frequently observed in patients with developmental disorders when compared with other groups. The exact mechanism of paradoxical reactions remains unclear. Most cases are idiosyncratic (Carissa et al. 2004). There is some evidence to suggest that these reactions may occur secondary to a genetic link, history of alcohol abuse, or psychological disturbances (Carissa et al. 2004; Short et al. 1987).

The reversal agent for benzodiazepines is flumazenil (Romazicon). It should be given via IV bolus, 0.2 mg (4–20 mcg/kg) at a rate of 0.2 mg/min. Titrate to patient response. The dentist may repeat at 20-minute intervals (Longmire & Seger 1993). Lack of patient response after cumulative dose of above implies that the major cause of sedation is unlikely to be benzodiazepines (Malamed 2010).

Sublingual or lingual injection of flumazenil is extremely controversial. Few studies have been performed to evaluate its efficacy (Hosaka et al. 2009). If multiple fluid boluses are given under the tongue, it could cause the tongue to swell and obstruct the airway (Hosaka et al. 2009).

## Opioids

Opioids, classified as strong analgesics, are administered for the relief of moderate to severe pain (Malamed 2010). Some anesthesia providers will select opioids as a preanesthetic drug because of their sedative, anti-anxiety, and analgesic properties. However, many will choose a sedative hypnotic or a benzodiazepine, unless severe pain is present. Opioid analgesics are divided into three categories: (1) opioid agonists, (2) opioid agonist-antagonists, and (3) opioid antagonists. Opioid agonists interact with the receptor (mu, kappa, sigma, and delta) and produce a physiologic change (Martin 1976; Phillips 1991). Opioid antagonists when bound produce no pharmacologic effect. Mixed agents produce characteristics of both. The receptor activated will determine the physiologic effect, which may include analgesia, sedation, euphoria, dysphoria, and respiratory depression (Phillips 1991).

A number of opioid agonists are used for sedation (moderate and deep) in dentistry. Meperidine (Demerol) was the most commonly used agent but it has been replaced by fentanyl and morphine, because of fewer side effects (Malamed 2010). Meperidine was found to have anti-cholinergic properties, which caused increased heart rate, decreased secretions, and localized histamine release (Pallasch 1973). These properties are not seen with fentanyl and morphine.

Morphine is the classic opioid by which other opioid agonists are compared for strength. It is not commonly used in outpatient IV moderate or deep sedation because of its relatively long duration of action. However, fentanyl, 100 times more potent than morphine, has a rapid onset and short duration of action, making it more desirable (Wedell & Hersh 1991). Analgesia and sedation are often immediate with IV fentanyl, although maximum effect is seen about 2–3 minutes later (Wedell & Hersh 1991).

Relative contraindications to use of opioid agonists include patients under the age of 2, pregnant patients, recent history of head trauma or CNS-related pathology, and MAOIs (monoamine oxidase inhibitors) within the past 14 days. Caution should be used in patients with renal or liver dysfunction (Malamed 2010). Opioids are also known to cause respiratory depression and stiff chest syndrome, which may result in hypoventilation and hypoxia. Therefore, the dentist must understand the concept of positive pressure ventilation if he or she is using opioids for sedation.

The reversal agent for opioid agonists is a pure opioid antagonist, naloxone hydrochloride (Narcan) (Martin 1976). Intravenous administration should result in rapid improvement of respiratory depression and reversal of the sedative effects. Naloxone's duration of action is about 20–30 minutes; therefore it is possible that if long-acting agonists were used patients may return to their sedated state. Reversals should be administered with care to persons with "known or suspected physical dependence on opioids" (Malamed 2010).

## Ketamine

Ketamine hydrochloride is a dissociative anesthetic (Reich & Silvay 1989). It produces a state in which the patient appears awake but unaware of or dissociated from the environment (Haas & Harper 1992). It is commonly administered to pediatric and older patients with developmental disorders. Routinely it is given with benzodiazepines to provide amnesia and analgesia. There is little to no respiratory depression as compared with benzodiazepines and opioids. Ketamine increases heart rate, blood pressure, and intra-cranial pressure and causes nystagmus and an incompetent gag reflex. Copious secretions result from ketamine administration and must be aggressively managed to prevent laryngospasm (Haas & Harper 1992).

Many experts believe dentists untrained in anesthesia should not administer ketamine (Malamed 2010). Different states have different guidelines for the use of ketamine for sedation in the dental office. There is no reversal agent for ketamine; therefore the dentist must be prepared to manage the patient and his or her level of sedation.

## Propofol

Propofol, nonbenzodiazepine, nonbarbiturate anesthetic, was originally designed as an induction agent for general anesthesia (Stuart Pharmaceuticals 1992). Recently propofol has received interest in outpatient venues because of it's sedation properties (MacKenzie & Grant 1987a, 1987b). When given at subhypnotic doses, it produces excellent sedation with minimal respiratory depression and a short recovery period (White & Negus 1991). Propofol is not recommended in pediatric patients and should only be administered by dentists with anesthesia training (Stuart Pharmaceuticals 1992).

## Chloral hydrate

Chloral hydrate is one of the oldest sedative hypnotics used in medicine and dentistry (Dionne et al. 2002). It is well absorbed when administered orally and distributes throughout, with good CNS uptake. It is metabolized rapidly to trichloroethanol (TCE) and trichloro-acetic acid (TCA). The sedative-hypnotic effects are caused by the activity of the TCE, which reaches peak plasma levels in 20–60 minutes, with prolonged plasma half-life estimated at 8 hours (Dionne et al. 2002).

Chloral hydrate has been a particularly popular drug for sedation and anxiety management in pediatric dentistry for many years (Dionne et al. 2006; Dionne 1998; Moore et al. 1984). Chloral hydrate is dosed on body weight, with a suggested range of 40–60 mg/kg to a maximum dose of 1 gram (Dionne et al. 2002; Dionne et al. 2006; Chloral Hydrate 2005; Noredenberg et al. 1971; Greenberg et al. 1993). Higher doses of chloral hydrate can cause GI irritation, including nausea and vomiting. Overdose with chloral hydrate includes life-threatening hypotension and respiratory arrest. Occasionally, chloral hydrate has been associated with arrhythmias (Dionne et al. 2006). There is no reversal agent for chloral hydrate (Moore et al. 1984).

## Antihistamines

Histamine (H1) blockers are used for treatment of allergy and for drying of secretions. However, a known side effect is CNS depression. The therapeutic window and margin of safety is high for antihistamines, making them popular in sedation dentistry (Malamed 2010). Hydroxyzine, a diphenylethane, is perhaps the most widely used antihistamine in pediatric dentistry (Wright & Chiasson 1973, 1987). It is used as a solo agent for management of children with mild to moderate fear. Combinations of hydroxyzine and other drugs such as meperidine, chloral hydrate, or midazolam are used for patients who require deeper levels of sedation (Torres-Perez et al. 2007). Fatal overdose with antihistamines is extremely uncommon and withdrawal from long-term use is not reported.

Antihistamines, like benzodiazepines, have been reported to cause paradoxical reactions in young children, elderly adults with genetic predisposition, alcoholics, and individuals with psychiatric and/or personality disorders (Carissa et al. 2004). Patients with developmental disorders are at higher risk for the development of comorbid psychiatric conditions, which predispose to idiosyncratic reactions (Antochi et al. 2003). Therefore, management of the psychiatric illness may reduce the severity of the paradoxical reaction.

# THE CONCEPT OF BALANCED ANESTHESIA

Balanced anesthesia is a technique in which two or more agents or methods of anesthesia produce a total desired effect. With a balanced approach, dentists are able to minimize patient risk and maximize patient comfort and safety. Balanced protocol requires individual assessment of the patient and the procedure in order to plan the office-based sedation. After the assessment, the dentist can choose the correct regimen, which perhaps is a mixture of several agents. Usually, balanced technique involves using a concurrent mixture of small amounts of several agents to summate in the desired level of sedation.

# MONITORING AND DOCUMENTATION

Studies show that routine application of cardiovascular and respiratory monitors enables the detection of subtle physiologic changes, which permits measures to be taken before there is a catastrophic event (Emergency Care Research Institute 1985). With that concept in mind the ASA developed guidelines for intra-operative monitoring as a national standard (Standards for Basic Intra-operative Monitoring 1986). As a rule of thumb, the deeper the sedation the more monitors should be used.

Below are excerpts from the American Academy of Pediatric Dentistry and American Academy of Pediatrics guidelines on monitoring sedation (AAPD 2007–2008):

## Moderate Sedation

### *Baseline*

Before administration of sedative medications, a baseline determination of vitals should be documented. For patients who are non-cooperative or are very upset, this may not be possible, and a note should be written to document behavior.

### *During the procedure*

The dentist should document the name, route, site, time of administration, and dosage of all drugs administered. There shall be continuous monitoring of oxygen saturation and heart rate and intermittent recording of respiratory rate and blood pressure; these should be recorded on a time-based record. Restraining devices should be checked to prevent airway obstruction or chest restriction. A functioning suction apparatus must be present.

### *After the procedure*

The patient who has received moderate sedation must be observed in a suitably equipped recovery facility (e.g., the facility must have functioning suction apparatus as well as the capacity to deliver more than 90% oxygen and positive pressure ventilation). The patient's vital signs should be recorded at specific intervals, until the patient meets discharge criteria or has completely returned to baseline status. If reversal agents have been used the patient will require a longer period of observation, because duration of the drugs administered may exceed the duration of the antagonist, which could lead to resedation.

### Deep sedation

The monitoring shall include all parameters as for moderate sedation. A competent provider shall observe the patient continuously. Vital signs, including oxygen saturation and heart rate, must be documented in a time-based record. Precordial stethoscope or capnography is encouraged for patients difficult to observe (AAPD 2007–2008; Hart et al. 1997).

## SPECIAL CONSIDERATIONS

- Physical restraint and mouth-stabilizing devices may be necessary to treat patients with a developmental disorder properly. The papoose board (Olympic Medical Corporation, Seattle) is an effective device to passively restrain the patient so that safe treatment may be accomplished (Figure 10.4). Note: *It is important not to overtighten the device over the patient's chest as it may restrict respiratory movement, which may already be decreased from sedative drugs* (Malamed 2010). Also, informed consent is mandatory for any type of physical restraint device. Use without consent could result in charges of assault and battery against the dentist (AAP 1992).

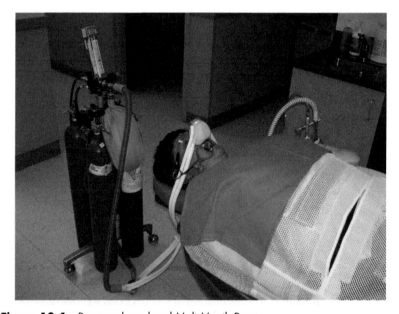

**Figure 10.4**  Papoose board and Molt Mouth Prop.

- Mouth-stabilizing devices are also available to aid the dentist in providing high-quality safe care. The most popular is a ratchet-type mouth prop (Molt Mouth Prop® Hu-Friedy, Chicago, IL). Once in the mouth, between the teeth, this device can be used to open the mouth to the desired level. Mouth props provide protection against the patient suddenly closing his or her mouth and improve access and visibility. Training for safe use is recommended. Periodontal teeth with excessive mobility and loose primary teeth in children are at risk for being knocked out and potentially aspirated. Mouth props also cause fatigue of facial/masticatory muscles and the temporomandibular joint. Therefore, care when using a prop should be exercised to avoid damage.
- Local anesthetic agents are cardiac depressants and may cause central nervous system excitation or depression (Moore 1999; AAPD 2007–2008). Drugs with similar mechanisms of action will have additive effects when administered in combination; therefore it is paramount not to exceed the maximum allowable safe dosage (Moore 1999; AAPD 2005). It is recommended that the dentist calculate the dose (mg/kg) prior to administration and administer slowly and with frequent aspiration to avoid possible intra-vascular injection (AAPD 2007–2008, 2005; Yagiela et al. 2004; Haas 2002; Malamed 2004).
- Phentolamine mesylate (OraVerse), a nonselective alpha-adrenergic blocking agent, is an approved reversal agent for local anesthetics with vasoconstrictors (Moore 2008). Phentolamine is specifically indicated for reversing soft tissue anesthesia, such as the lip, tongue, and buccal mucosa. Prolonged soft tissue anesthesia can result in inadvertent biting, causing severe injury. Therefore, reducing the duration of posttreatment anesthesia may reduce the posttreatment injury due to biting (Tavares et al. 2008). The greatest benefit from reversal may be seen in children and patients with developmental disorders (Tavares et al. 2008). Phentolamine is not indicated for children younger than 6 years of age or less than 15 kg (33 lbs.) (OraVerse 2009).

# EMERGENCIES

The standard of care for emergencies arising as part of sedation is the same as any medical emergency. The dentist needs to recognize there is a problem and quickly address the issue. Dentists who have training in local anesthesia alone see syncope as a medical emergency. Dentists who administer sedation may occasionally experience unconsciousness or apnea. They should be prepared to treat the patient seamlessly. As with deep sedation and general anesthesia the goal is an unconscious patient, so apnea is a routine occurrence and would not be considered an emergency. What may be an emergency to one provider may be a normal occurrence to another (Malamed 2010).

The dentist should always evaluate risks versus benefits specific to the patient with a developmental disorder. In an effort to minimize sedation-related events it is recommended that the dentist have a comfortable relationship with the patient and caregivers, use familiar drugs and techniques, limit the use to patients who require them, have a comprehensive preop evaluation, and have continuous monitoring. An emergency system should be in place with trained personnel who can follow the protocol. All high-risk patients should be treated in a hospital setting (AAPD 2007–2008).

The selection of emergency drugs and armamentarium must be based on the training and background of the dentist who is responsible for its use. Regardless, it is vital that the dentist is familiar with indications, contraindications, dosages, and method of administration of emergency drugs and be able to correctly operate any available equipment.

Potential emergency situations include: (Malamed 2010)

1. Overdose.
2. Allergic reactions.
3. Hypotension/hypertension.
4. Cardiac arrhythmias.
5. Angina pectoris/acute myocardial infarction.
6. Airway obstruction.
7. Laryngospasm.
8. Foreign body aspiration.
9. Hyperventilation.
10. Respiratory depression.
11. Seizures.
12. Hypoglycemia.
13. Syncope.

Once an emergency has been identified, it is important that everyone remains calm, then assesses the situation, followed by the PABCs (Malamed 2010):

P = Position: always position patient appropriately.
A = Airway: assess to see if patient's airway is patent.
B = Breathing: determine if patient is breathing.
C = Circulation: check to see if there is a pulse.
D = Definitive care: may include activation of EMS and establishing IV access.
E = Electricity: assess need.

Note: Respiratory events are the most common cause of sedation-related emergencies in pediatric patients with developmental disorders and normal cardiac function. Therefore, the dentist needs to be skilled in airway management and understand the concept of positive pressure ventilation (bag-valve-mask) with 100% oxygen. If airway issues are not addressed, the respiratory event could result in cardiac arrest.

## CLOSING COMMENTS

There are many techniques available to dentists and dental hygienists to control pain and anxiety in patients with a developmental disorder. The method of choice should be based on office preparedness, the provider's comfort level, and training. There is no one correct method for each dentist or patient. Remember there is no panacea, nor is one technique going to work for every patient. Therefore, having multiple options for sedation will decrease your risk of failure.

### Disclaimer

- This chapter is not intended to make you proficient in sedation for the patient with a developmental disorder.
- Information presented is based on Guidelines from the American Academy of Pediatric Dentistry, American Dental Association, American Academy of Pediatrics, and the American Society of Anesthesiologists.
- The provider must know their state guidelines and regulations before administering any type of sedation.

## REFERENCES

Alcaino EA. (2000). Conscious sedation in paediatric dentistry: Current philosophies and techniques. Annals of the Royal Australasian College of Dental Surgeons 15:206–210.

American Academy of Pediatric Dentistry (AAPD). (2005). Guideline on appropriate use of local anesthesia for pediatric dental patients. *Pediatric Dentistry* 27(suppl):101–106.

———. (2007–2008). Guidelines for monitoring and management of pediatric patients during and after sedation for diagnostic and therapeutic procedures. *Pediatric Dentistry* 29(7 Reference Manual):134–151.

American Academy of Pediatrics (AAP) Committee on Child Abuse and Neglect. (1992). Behavior management of pediatric dental patients. *Pediatrics* 90:651.

American Dental Association (ADA), Council on Dental Education. (2007a). Guidelines for the use of sedation and general anesthesia by dentists. As adopted by the October 2007 *American Dental Association's House of Delegates*, Chicago, IL.

———. (2007b). Guidelines for teaching pain control and sedation in dentists and dental students. As adopted by the October 2007 *American Dental Association's House of Delegates*, Chicago, IL.

American Heart Association (AHA). (2002). *Pediatric Advanced Life Support Provider Manual*. Dallas: American Heart Association.

American Society of Anesthesiologists (ASA). (1963). New classification of physical status. *Anesthesiology* 24:111.

———. (2002). Task Force on Sedation and Analgesia by Non-Anesthesiologists: Practice guidelines for sedation and analgesia by non-anesthesiologists. *Anesthesiology* 96:1004–1017.

Antochi R, Stavarkaki C, Emery PC. (2003). Psychopharmacological treatments in persons with dual diagnosis of psychiatric disorders and developmental disabilities. *Postgraduate Medical Journal* 79:139–146.

Carissa E, Mancuso CE, Tanzi MG, Gabay, M. (2004). Paradoxical reactions to benzodiazepines: Literature review and treatment options. *Pharmacotherapy* 24(9):1177–1185.

Carr MP, Horton JE. (2001). Clinical evaluation and comparison of 2 topical anesthetics for pain caused by needle sticks and scaling and root planning. *Journal of Periodontology* 72(4):479–484.

Chloral Hydrate Oral Solution. (2005). *Package insert. Vintage Pharmaceuticals, LLC, Huntsville, AL.*

Clark MS, Brunick AL. (1999). *Handbook of Nitrous Oxide and Oxygen Sedation*, 2nd ed. St. Louis: Mosby.

———. (2008). *Handbook of Nitrous Oxide and Oxygen Sedation*, 3rd ed. St. Louis: Mosby.

Conner JT, Katz RL, Pagano RR, et al. (1978). Midazolam for intravenous surgical premedication, and induction of general anesthesia. *Anesthesia/Analgesia* 57:1.

Cote CJ, Notterman DS, Karl HW, Weinberg JA, McClosekey C. (2000). Adverse sedation events in pediatrics: A critical incident analysis of contributory factors. *Pediatrics* 105:805–814.

Cravero JP, Blike GT. (2004). Review of pediatric sedation. *Anesthesia & Analgesia* 99:1355–1364.

Deshpande JK, Tobias JD, eds. (1996). *The Pediatric Pain Handbook.* St. Louis: Mosby.

Dionne R. (1998). Oral sedation. *Compendium of Continuing Education in Dentistry* 19:868–870.

Dionne R, Phero J, Becker D. (2002). *Management of Pain and Anxiety in the Dental Office.* Philadelphia: W.B. Saunders, pp. 230–231, 306–310.

Dionne R, Yagiela J, Cote C, Donaldson M, Edwards M, Greenblatt D, Haas D, Malviya S, Milgrom P, Moore P, Shampaine G, Silverman M, Williams R, Wilson S. (2006). Balancing efficacy and safety in the use of oral sedation in dental outpatients. *Journal of the American Dental Association* 137(4):502–513.

Douglas BL. (1958). A re-evaluation of Guedel's stages of anesthesia: With particular reference to the ambulatory dental patient. *Journal of the American Dental Society of Anesthesiology* 5(1):11–14.

Emergency Care Research Institute. (1985). Death during general anesthesia. *Journal of Health Care Technology* 1:155.

Feld LH, Negus JB, White PF. (1990). Oral midazolam preanesthetic drug in pediatric outpatients. *Anesthesiology* 73:831.

Flaitz CM, Nowak AJ, Hicks MJ. (1986). Evaluation of aneterograde amnesic effect of rectally administered diazepam in the sedated pedodontic patient. *Journal of Dentistry for Children* 53:17.

Fleisher LA. (2005). Risk of anesthesia. In R.D. Miller, L.A. Fleisher, R.A. Johns (Eds.), *Miller's Anesthesia*, 6th ed. New York: Churchill Livingstone.

Fukota O, Braham RL, Yanase H, et al. (1993). The sedative effect of intranasal midazolam administration in the dental treatment of patients with mental disabilities. Part 1: The effect of 0.2 mg/kg dose. *Journal of Clinical Pediatric Dentistry* 17(4):231–237.

Fuks AB, Kaufman E, Ram D, et al. (1994). Assessment of two doses of intranasal midazolam for sedation of pediatric dental patients. *Pediatric Dentistry* 16(4):301–305.

Giovannitti JA, Moore PA. (2011). Sedative-hypnotics, antianxiety drugs, and centrally acting muscle relaxants. In J. Yagiela, F. Dowd, B. Johnson, A. Mariotti, E. Neidle (Eds.), *Pharmacology and Therapeutics for Dentistry*, 6th ed. (pp. 188–211). St. Louis: Mosby Elsevier.

Greenberg SB, Faerber EN, Aspinall CL, et al. (1993). High dose chloral hydrate sedation for children undergoing MR imaging: Safety and efficacy in relation to age. *American Journal of Roentgenology* 161:639–641.

Haas DA. (2002). An update on local anesthetics in dentistry. *Journal of Canadian Dental Association* 68:546–551.

Haas DA, Harper DG. (1992). Ketamine: A review of its pharmacologic properties and use in ambulatory anesthesia. *Anesthesia Progress* 39:61.

Harrison-Calmes S. (2002). Arthur Guedel, M.D., and the eye signs of anesthesia. *ASA Newsletter* 66(9).

Hart LS, Berns SD, Houck CS, Boenning DS. (1997). The value of end-tidal $CO_2$ monitoring when comparing three methods of conscious sedation for children undergoing painful procedure in the emergency department. *Pediatric Emergency Care* 13:189–193.

Hennesy MJ, Kirby KC, Montgomery IM. (1991). Comparison of the amnesic effects of midazolam and diazepam. *Psychopharmacology* 103:545.

Hoffman GM, Nowakowski R, Troshynski TJ, Bernes RJ, Weisman SJ. (2002). Risk reduction in pediatric procedural sedation by application of an American Academy of Pediatrics/American Society of Anesthesiologists process model. *Pediatrics* 109:236–243.

Hosaka K, Jackson D, Pickrell JE, Heima M, Milgrom P. (2009). Flumazenil reversal of sublingual triazolam: A randomized clinical trial. *Journal of the American Dental Association* 140(5):559–566.

Jastak JT, Donaldson D. (1991). Nitrous oxide. *Anesthesia Progress* 38:172.

Jastak JT, Orendruff D. (1975). Recovery from nitrous sedation. *Anesthesia Progress* 22:113–116.

Jensen B, Matsson L. (2001). Benzodiazepines in child dental care: A survey of its use among general practitioners and paediatric dentists in Sweden. *Swedish Dental Journal* 25(1):31–38.

Kennedy RM, Luchman JD. (1999). The ouchless emergency department. Getting closer: Advances in decreasing distress during painful procedures in the emergency department. *Pediatric Clinics of North America* 46:1215–1247.

Krauss B, Green SM. (2006). Procedural sedation and analgesia in children. *Lancet* 367:766–780.

Lagasse RS. (2002). Anesthesia safety: Model of myth? A review of published literature and analysis of current original data. *Anesthesiology* 97: 1609–1617.

Lam C, Udin RD, Malamed SF, et al. (2005). Midazolam premedication in children: A pilot study comparing intramuscular and intranasal administration. *Anesthesia Progress* 52(2):56–61.

Longmire AW, Seger DL. (1993). Topics in clinical pharmacology; Flumazenil, a benzodiazepine antagonist. *American Journal of Medical Science* 306:49.

Mace SE, Barata IA, Cravero JP, et al. (2004). Clinical policy: Evidence-based approach to pharmacologic agents used in pediatric sedation and analgesia in the emergency department. *Annals of Emergency Medicine* 44:342–377.

MacKenzie N, Grant IS. (1987a). Propofol for intravenous sedation. *Anaesthesia* 42:3.

———. (1987b). Propofol infusion for sedation in the intensive care unit. *British Medical Journal* 294:774.

Malamed SF. (2004). Local anesthetic considerations in dental specialties. In *Handbook of Local Anesthesia*, 5th ed. (pp. 269, 274–275). St. Louis: Mosby.

———. (2010). *Sedation: A Guide to Patient Management*, 5th ed. St. Louis: Mosby Elsevier.

Malviya S, Naughton NN, Tremper KT, eds. (2001). *Sedation Analgesia for Diagnostic and Therapeutic Procedures*. Totowa, NJ: Humana Press.

Malviya S, Vopel-Lewis T, Tait AR. (1997). Adverse events and risk factors associated with the sedation of children by non-anesthesiologist. *Anesthesia & Analgesia* 85:1207–1213.

Martin WR. (1976). Naloxone. *Annals of Internal Medicine* 85:765.

Maxwell LG, Yaster M. (1996). The myth of conscious sedation. *Archives of Pediatric & Adolescent Medicine* 150:605–607.

Mitchell AA, Louik C, Lacouture P, Slone D, Goldman P, Shapiro S. (1982). Risks to children from computed tomographic scan premedication. *Journal of the American Medical Association* 247:2385–2388.

Moore PA. (1999). Adverse drug interactions in dental practice: Interactions associated with local anesthetics, sedatives and anxiolytics: Part IV of a series. *Journal of the American Dental Association* 130:541–554.

———. (2008). Pharmacokinetics of lidocaine with epinephrine following local anesthesia reversal with phentolamine mesylate. *Anesthesia Progress* 55:40–48.

Moore PA, Mickey EA, Hargreaves JA, Needleman HL. (1984). Sedation in pediatric dentistry: A practical assessment procedure. *Journal of the American Dental Association* 109:564–569.

Newton JT, Shah S, Patel H, Sturmey P. (2003). Non-pharmacological approaches to behavior management in children. *Dental Update* 30:194–199.

Noredenberg A, Dalisle G, Izukawa T. (1971). Cardiac arrhythmias in a child due to chloral hydrate ingestion. *Pediatrics* 47:134.

OraVerse. (2009). Package insert. Accessed August 20, 2009, from http://www.novalar.com/assets/pdf/package_insert_jan09.pdf.

Pallasch TJ. (1973). *Clinical Drug Therapy in Dental Practice*. Philadelphia: Lea & Febiger.

Parnis SJ, Foate JA, Vander Wlath JH, et al. (1992). Oral midazolam is an effective premedicant for children having day-care. *Anaesthesia and Intensive Care* 20:9–14.

Phillips WJ. (1991). Central nervous system pain receptors. In R. J. Faust (Ed.), *Anesthesiology Review*. New York: Churchill Livingstone.

Reich DL, Silvay G. (1989). "Ketamine: An update on the first twenty-five years of clinical experience." *Canadian Journal of Anesthesia* 36:186.

Short TG, Forrest P, Galletly DC. (1987). Paradoxical reactions to benzodiazepines: A genetically determined phenomenon? *Anaesthesia and Intensive Care* 15:330–345.

Sinner B, Graf BM. (2008). Ketamine. *Handbook of Experimental Pharmacology* 182:313–333.

Standards for Basic Intra-operative Monitoring. (1986). *ASA Newsletter* 50:13.

Stuart Pharmaceuticals: Diprivan. (1992). *Package insert*. Wilmington, Delaware.

Tavares M, Goodson M, Studen-Pavlovich D, Yagiela J, Navalta L, Rogy S, Rutherford B, Gordon S, Papas A. (2008). Reversal of soft tissue local anesthesia with phentolamine mesylate in pediatric patients. *Journal of the American Dental Association* 139:1095–1105.

Torres-Perez J, Tapia-Garcia I, Rosales-Berber MA, et al. (2007). Comparison of three conscious sedation regimens for pediatric dental patients. *Journal of Clinical Pediatric Dentistry* 31(3):183–186.

Walbergh EJ, Wills RJ, Eckhert J. (1991). Plasma concentrations of midazolam in children following intranasal administration. *Anesthesiology* 74:233.

Wedell D, Hersh EV. (1991). A review of the opioid analgesics, fentanyl, alfentanil and sufentanil. *Compendium* 12:184–187.

Weinbroum AA, Szold O, Ogorek D, Flasishon R. (2001). The midazolam-induced paradox phenomenon is reversible by flumazenil: Epidemiology, patient characteristics and review of the literature. *European Journal of Anaesthesiology* 18:789–797.

White PF, Negus JB. (1991). Sedative infusions during local or intravenous regional anesthesia: A comparison of propofol and midazolam. *Journal of Clinical Anesthesia* 3:32.

Wright GZ, Chiasson RC. (1973). Current premedicating trends in pedodontics. *Journal of Children's Dentistry* 40:185.

———. (1987). The use of sedation drugs by Canadian pediatric dentists. *Pediatric Dentistry* 9:308.

Yagiela JA, Neidle EA, Dowd FJ. (2004). Local anesthetics. In *Pharmacology and Therapeutics for Dentistry* (pp. 251–270). Philadelphia: Elsevier Health Science.

Yaster M, Krane EJ, Kaplan RF, Cote CJ, Lappe DG, eds. (1997). *Pediatric Pain Management and Sedation Handbook*. St. Louis: Mosby.

# 11

# Hospital dentistry/general anesthesia

## Allen Wong, DDS, EdD, DABSCD

## WHEN IS IT NECESSARY?

The continuum of dental care delivery ranges from being treated in a routine dental office setting with no anesthesia to being treated at a hospital with general anesthesia. The purpose of this chapter is to help demystify the question of "When is general anesthesia necessary?" by reviewing the concerns for the patient who is being considered for general anesthesia from a medical and dental perspective.

General anesthesia is considered when the most conservative options have been explored and the benefits of anesthesia outweigh the risks. Safety for the patient and dental team along with consideration of overall health benefits are the focus of the decision. General anesthesia is usually performed either in a surgery center or hospital. Hospitals have the advantage of providing an option of inpatient or outpatient settings, whereas most surgery centers offer only outpatient care. Outpatient surgery is common for most patients unless significant medical concerns or chronic medical conditions are in question. Not all hospitals have dental services or have dentists with operating room privileges. There is rapid growth in the need for safe and high-quality office-based anesthesia. To meet these needs, a special set of skills is required, which may require expanded exposure and experience during training (Perrott 2008; Wong 2010).

There should be a justified medical and dental rationale for seeking dentistry under general anesthesia. Medical complexity, physical limitations,

*Treating the Dental Patient with a Developmental Disorder*, First Edition.
Edited by Karen A. Raposa and Steven P. Perlman.
© 2012 John Wiley & Sons, Inc. Published 2012 by John Wiley & Sons, Inc.

and neurologic and psychological considerations are some of the common reasons for admissions. A suspicion of dental pathology that may exist or a prolonged period of undetermined oral condition would be a reasonable concern.

There is still a great need for more studies to assess the risk versus benefit for patients with developmental disorders and to stratify such risk in order to assist care providers in decision making as well as in sharing such risk concerns with patients, caretakers, and guardians (Messieha 2009). Most dental cases seen in the operating room are considered elective. The dental case only becomes emergent when the dental pathology is severe and the spread of infection is imminent and negatively contributes to the patient's health and is possibly life threatening.

The term "hospital dentistry" is described as dentists that perform routine dentistry in a hospital clinic, dentists that consult bedside, and/or dentists that provide dentistry in the operating room.

In this chapter, we will focus on the definition of the term "hospital dentistry" as requiring general anesthesia in the operating room. The dental services that hospital dentistry provides can range from only extractions to all phases of dental disciplines including limited orthodontics, fixed prosthodontics, and endodontics. If planned in advance, additional necessary medical procedures can be combined during the time of general anesthesia. Routine medical procedures such as blood work, chemistry levels, ear exams, eye exams, gynecological exams, chest x-rays, cardioversions (shocking of the heart to return to normal synchronization), and podiatric procedures are just some of the medical procedures that can be done if the facility and the physician services are offered for the patient who cannot cooperate. It would be best to explore these options well in advance.

## MEDICAL NECESSITY

Medical necessity can encompass acquired and congenital medical diagnoses, physical limitations, emotional limitations, and physical limitations and/or developmental disabilities that make cooperation difficult. It is important to emphasize that not all patients with developmental disabilities (DDs), neurodevelopmental disabilities (NDs), or intellectual disabilities (IDs) need to be seen in the hospital. Once convinced that it would be safer to treat the patient under general anesthesia, the dentist concentrates on the dental needs, the intricacy of the procedures, and the amount of work that needs to be done. The choices of the appropriate hospital and anesthesia are then considered and selected.

For patients who cannot verbalize their oral condition, they may exhibit their concerns in changes in mood or changes in eating patterns. This patient may be more aggressive or more guarded in an area where there is some dental pathology. Fevers of unknown origin, bleeding from the mouth, or swelling of the face could be clues to an oral concern.

A preliminary oral pathology list is derived and carefully evaluated. An important aspect of diagnosing pathology is the question of etiology with respect to physiologic and biologic factors. How did the cavity or concern develop? Was it from neglect, or did the medical diagnosis/medications accentuate the spread of dental caries and periodontitis?

One of the important concerns is the oral condition secondary to medication and the treatment of the medical diagnosis. What predisposing factors can be mitigated to improve the final outcome? The caries risk assessment and the strategies for lowering risk are essential so that proper choices in treatment options are considered.

# DENTAL NECESSITY

Ideally, a complete oral examination and dental radiographs are obtained, if the patient can tolerate them, prior to the operation. In cases where the patient is not cooperative for evaluation, oral sedation may be considered. Oral sedation should be discussed with the primary care provider if the patient is taking multiple medications. Patients with acute symptoms such as pain, swelling, and bleeding should have a greater urgency when scheduling as opposed to a case for a routine checkup. The amount of dental work and sophistication of the work needed will affect the amount of time needed and requested in the operating room (Wong 2009).

There are no absolute limitations to how many times a person can have general anesthesia, but it would be advised to lessen the risk of anesthesia by limiting the need for return hospital visits.

For cases that cannot be evaluated properly without deep sedation, the option could be to have sedation for the sole purpose of examination and radiographs and emergent treatment for suspected pathology, with another visit for comprehensive treatment. Having multiple surgeries increases the cost of the hospital cases as well as repeats the anesthesia risks. Of course, there are times when it is necessary to have additional surgery dates if the case is too complex, too lengthy, or additional follow-up procedures are indicated.

A hospital dentist is able to only perform procedures he or she has requested (and has privileges for) and has proven competence to perform. Should procedures be requested or needed that the dentist cannot perform, the dentist must decide whether another dentist with such privileges may be needed to complete the procedure.

Cases can be scheduled either on a first-come, first-served basis or by a triaged system (ranking of needs through clinical identifiers) that schedules based upon urgency (Wong 2009).

# PATIENT ABILITY

Assessing the patient's understanding of his or her role and the importance of oral care is crucial to the overall treatment plan (Waldman et al. 2008). The patient who is aggressive and will not allow a caregiver or help in his or her oral hygiene does not give great promise for elaborate dental restorative options. A person who is physically unable to brush his or her teeth or floss is also one that does not lead the dentist toward complex dental restorations. Basically, cooperation and attention to care are key to a degree of dental work provided and its longevity. The patient who has physical limitations such as dexterity, limited mouth opening, and difficultly expectorating has additional considerations in terms of treatment options. Some of the challenges can be mitigated with a thorough caregiver's attention and help.

# CAREGIVER ABILITY

For those patients who cannot physically maintain their oral health and are dependent upon their caregiver, there are additional concerns. The caregiver must have the understanding and the willingness to follow instructions for a good oral health care regime. If the caregiver is not following the instructions carefully, premature tooth loss can be a consequence.

Education and training for caregivers should become a standard of care early in the first year of life for any child with a developmental delay or any person, regardless of age, who experiences an illness or event that compromises his or her ability to provide self–oral health care (Ferguson & Cinotti 2009). Therefore, the caregiver's ability to properly care for the mouth is crucial for the overall success of the dental treatment. It is in essence oral care therapy with the emphasis on remineralization of teeth.

# GOAL

The overarching goal of hospital dentistry should be to get the patient restored to optimal oral health and then be followed up with a preventive dentistry plan. The patient who needs hospital dentistry most likely has a high caries risk factor. If the dental caries risk factors are not addressed, the likelihood that the patient would be seen again soon for additional procedures, namely extractions, is great.

When the protective actions of saliva are impaired, the buffering capacity of saliva is reduced and it is unable to adequately neutralize the acids in the mouth. The quality and quantity of saliva is key to minimizing dental caries and extending the life of dental restorations (Featherstone 2004).

Once the hospital dentistry case is completed, the oral pathologies of caries and periodontitis should be corrected and the negative dental biofilm (bacterial plaque) should be neutralized. The hospital dental procedure is just a step in the healing process; the importance of follow-up care cannot be understated. If the biofilm is properly restored to health and a remineralization strategy is employed, the patient can lower his or her caries risk significantly for a longer period of time. Oral biofilm can be treated with intra-operative oral preparations of iodine solution or chlorhexidine topically brushed if the patient is not allergic to the solutions. While the patient is under sedation, the surface contact time for which the solution remains in the mouth is maximized because the patient cannot taste or react.

The use of sugar alcohols, povidone-iodine, delmopinol, triclosan, and chlorhexidine may modulate the caries process. In addition, studies involving probiotics and molecular genetics have provided results showing that these methods can replace and displace cariogenic bacteria with noncariogenic bacteria, while maintaining normal oral homeostasis (Garcia-Godoy & Hicks 2008; Slots 2002).

## MEDICAL ASSESSMENT

The patient may either have an acquired or congenital medical diagnosis. The overall health of the patient determines the level of hospital care needed. It is not uncommon to have a patient with multiple diagnoses. Anesthesia risks are mostly either a heart or lung issue. The anesthesiologist who performs the surgery should have some experience with patients with developmental disabilities, as many have medical comorbid conditions yet to be evaluated (Waldman et al. 2009). The systemic health of the patient is qualified in a classification developed by the American Society of Anesthesiologists (ASA). The classification goes from ASA 1 to ASA 6, with one being healthy and the greater the number, the less healthy. The oral systemic connection cannot be denied, and patients with special needs often have symptoms of gastric reflux (GERD), cardiovascular concerns, and potential medication interactions.

The primary care provider should assess the patient's health for tolerance to general anesthesia. The assessment is called a history and physical for clearance for general anesthesia and focuses on the cardiovascular and pulmonary functions, as well as any other medical conditions that may contribute to care. Depending on the patient's age and medical diagnoses, certain preoperative tests may be necessary. Both the assessment and tests should be done as close to the day of the procedure as possible, but not so early that the report is unavailable or corrections to a medical condition cannot be made a few days before the actual procedure. In some circumstances, a specialist may be needed, thus requiring additional time for the clearance.

For more involved medical conditions, a preoperative evaluation for general anesthesia would be advised from the anesthesia department prior to scheduling a case.

# MEDICATIONS

A thorough review of the patient's medication will need to be confirmed with his or her physician. Seldom will there be modification to daily medication regime. Drug allergies should be thoroughly reviewed and alternative medicines such as analgesics and antibiotics should be agreed upon. Many medications prescribed may cause or contribute to salivary hypofunction (xerostomia or dry mouth) or hyperacidity of the oral environment or impair the buffering capacity of saliva. Saliva produced from salivary glands is the natural protective fluid to protect teeth from demineralization. The mouth has many major and minor salivary glands and the quality and quantity (flow rate) is important to effectively protect teeth.

For patients with a tendency toward an acidic oral environment and/or to lessen salivary flow, attention should be concentrated on improving the salivary flow and salivary chemistry.

All medications including herbal should be taken to the appointment to be reviewed.

# ANESTHESIOLOGICAL ASSESSMENT

An anesthesiologist or qualified nurse anesthetist must assess the cooperation level of the patient for following verbal instructions, attaining an intravenous catheter, and the patient's baseline condition. The ultimate goal is to safely administer medications to the patient to allow a smooth induction and placement of a breathing tube through the nose or mouth. In order to administer medication, the IV site should be able to be visualized and palpable. The neck extension should be comfortable in a slight hyperextension with no loose teeth and a mouth opening that can allow visualization of the throat. In cases where there is restriction in the nose, mouth, or throat, the fiber-optic instrument approach may be used.

In anesthesiology, the Mallampati score, also Mallampati classification, is used to predict the ease of intubation. It is determined by looking at the anatomy of the oral cavity; specifically, it is based on the visibility of the base of the uvula, faucial pillars (the arches in front of and behind the tonsils) and soft palate. Scoring may be done with or without phonation. A high Mallampati score (class 4) is associated with more difficult intubation, as well as a higher incidence of sleep apnea.

Scoring is as follows:

Class 1: full visibility of tonsils, uvula, and soft palate.

Class 2: visibility of hard and soft palate, upper portion of tonsils, and uvula.

Class 3: soft and hard palate and base of the uvula are visible.

Class 4: only hard palate visible (Mallampati et al. 1985; Nuckton et al. 2006).

The greater the classification, the more preparations are needed for a difficult airway. Time is of the essence during the intubation phase.

## LIMITATIONS OF HOSPITALS

Many hospitals can accommodate both children and adults. Patients with more complex medical conditions may require a hospital that has the ability to manage overnight telemetry. The highest of medical risks would require an intensive care unit. Pediatric ICUs are not always at every hospital. For hospitals and ambulatory care hospitals without ICUs or that do not have the ability to conduct overnight observation of a patient, there is usually an arrangement with a local hospital to manage the patient. Patients with acute distress may be seen for treatment of the acute problem only. Less time is needed in the schedule and therefore it is easier to add to a schedule for "emergent" cases. A "dental emergency" is defined as extreme pain, swelling, and/or bleeding or any combination of the three.

There are three financial considerations for the patient: (1) hospital fees, (2) anesthesiologist fees, and (3) dental fees. The patient is ultimately responsible for the portions not covered by medical and dental insurances. A preestimate is advised, as medical insurance may have stipulations to the hospital coverage when it is related to dentistry.

Most hospitals have compensation concerns for their facility charges when dental procedures are done in the operating room. Facility charges cover the hospital bed upon admission, the preoperative preparation of the nursing staff, the necessary supplies (for admission and the anesthesia area), and the postoperative recovery room and staffing. Some medical insurance will not cover a patient for dental services in the operating room solely for convenience. The hospital needs to communicate to medical insurance that the patient is being seen due to chronic medical diagnosis, the procedure happens to be dental in nature, and the patient cannot be seen safely in a routine setting. The anesthesiologist will bill the medical insurance for his or her services. Dental procedures are billed to the dental insurances in the usual fashion.

If there are concerns, the hospital has a billing/finance department that can help with clarifying medical coverage and payment options.

## WORKING WITH PRIMARY CARE PHYSICIANS

It cannot be stressed enough that the whole process is a team approach. It is imperative that the primary care physician who is most familiar with the patient be involved. The physician and dentist should be on the same page as they plan for the patient's hospital dentistry experience. All concerns should be adequately addressed so that the patient is prepared well for surgery. In some cases, additional medical information can be coordinated with the dental surgeon. Some such examples are blood work and physical examinations (ob/gyn, eye, ear, feet, cardiac tests, etc.). The primary care physician would make the request and help to attain the physician for the additional physical exams.

## SPECIAL CIRCUMSTANCES: PHYSICAL LIMITATIONS

- Weight limitation—patients with significant weight and immobility may require a Hoyer lift to move the patient from gurney to operating table and an extra-wide wheelchair for transport use. Due to the limited amount of supplies, there may be a need to request these items in advance.
- Cardiac monitoring—pacemaker users may require advanced scheduling to assure that a specialist or product representative be av ailable for settings of the device.
- Questionable cardiac conditions may require a portable EKG in the operating room for uncooperative patients.
- Imaging/x-rays (nondental) in the operating room while under sedation—chest x-rays for patients with question of cardiac anomaly or suspected aspiration (water or foreign object in the lung) during or postoperative may be necessary. Most hospitals have radiology departments that have the availability but may need to be scheduled. Head and skull films may be arranged for patients unable to take oral radiographs due to physical limitations or questions of anatomical structure. Coordinated CT scans/MRIs may sometimes be possible.

## PREOPERATIVE PLANNING

Once the decision has been made for hospital dentistry, it is necessary to prepare the patient for the experience. Desensitization is an important part of the procedure to better prepare the patient and the caregivers. The day of surgery is not the day for additional stress. Depending on the patient's cooperation level, the desensitization may be as simple as discussing the procedure and the course of the hospital stay. Some patients may need a brief tour of the facility and review of the hospital procedures to feel more comfortable prior to the day of surgery.

The goal on the day of surgery is for the patient to have an intravenous catheter placed. If the patient is more relaxed, many times he or she is able to tolerate the catheterization with good rapport. If the patient is more apprehensive and less cooperative, a discussion with his or her primary care physician for oral premedication may be in order prior to arrival at the hospital. For some individuals, picture books of the procedures may help to introduce the patient to what to expect.

As some anxiolytic premedications may cause a paradoxical (opposite) reaction such as excitation instead of sedation, a test dosage at home may be useful strategy.

As soon as the patient arrives, the routine baseline information of height, weight, blood pressure, review of medications, empty stomach status, and consents are reviewed. It is advised that the patient come in clothing that can be easily removed, and he or she should be prepared to have monitors placed on the finger for pulse oximetry, on the arm for blood pressure, and EKG stickers on the chest.

Once consent is confirmed, an intravenous catheter is inserted, if the patient tolerates it. If patient is too anxious, a sedative is given after the anesthesiologist agrees on the safety, either an oral route (pill or liquid), an injection, or a mask-induction approach.

Parents or caregivers are sometimes allowed to accompany the patient when the surgeon and anesthesiologist feel it is a benefit for the patient. There are times when the emotion of the parent/caregiver is a distraction for the patient and the process.

After the patient has received enough medication to cause anesthesia, a breathing tube is gently placed in either the nose or mouth depending on need and safety. If needed, dental radiographs are taken after a lead shield is placed over the thyroid and chest area.

An examination is then performed with a list of pathologies and dental treatment options considered. A gauze throat pack is gently placed in the back of the mouth to minimize aspiration of fluids and foreign objects into the lungs. The mouth is prepared with anti-microbial solution to lower the bacterial count and destroy the biofilm.

If there are restorations considered, the mouth should be thoroughly debrided (cleaned) before the restoration phase. Restorations may be as simple as sealants and as involved as root canals. The dental material choice would be determined with a consideration for the patient's dental caries risk. The systematic approach in determining caries risk known as Caries Management by Risk Assessment (CAMBRA) or Caries Risk Assessment or Caries Assessment Tools helps to make a logical choice of dental materials, prevention strategies, and follow-up intervals. For online journal information about CAMBRA, visit http://www.cdafoundation.org/who_we_are/publications.../cda_journal_october_2007, or http://www.cdafoundation.org/who_we_are/publication.../cda_journal_november_2007

The choice for the high caries patient should be to have the oral biofilm controlled with anti-microbials if needed and the consideration for filling material ought to be anti-cariogenic or cariostatic. The materials that resist caries are either glass ionomers for their fluoride release or alloys for their corrosion seal of margins. Composite restorations require a patient with healthy biofilm in order for the resins to be resistant to recurrent caries. Once the biofilm is controlled and the acid levels of the mouth are neutralized, it is possible to help remineralize teeth that have exhibited demineralization. Early signs of demineralization may be seen clinically and appear as white spots or frosted lesions on teeth. The concept of remineralization is useful on teeth that begin to exhibit signs of demineralization. Remineralization requires fluoride, calcium, and phosphate in a neutral environment. In healthy saliva, fluoride, calcium, and phosphate are present and available to remineralize. Additional fluoride, calcium, and phosphate may improve remineralization uptake. Fluoride can be applied in many forms. Fluoride is available in varnishes, rinses, toothpaste, foam, fluoride trays, and glass ionomer products. Remineralization is most effective in a neutral pH environment (Weintraub et al. 2006).

## SOFT TISSUE REPAIR

When oral surgery is necessary for soft tissue repair, it should be treated as a surgical intervention with the goal of primary closure (minimal gap between tissue) to minimize potential dry socket "postextraction alveolitis" secondary to food or finger trauma. To lessen the patient's stress of removing silk sutures, resorbable sutures are encouraged.

## OCCLUSION

Occlusion can only be checked when nasal intubation is the route for general anesthesia. Should the patient have an endotracheal tube from the mouth, the need for careful adjustment of occlusion is essential. Local anesthesia may be infiltrated in areas of suspected concerns of potential operative and postoperative discomfort.

## SOFT TISSUE TRAUMA

The goal of postoperative condition is patient comfort and analgesics with minimal narcotics. Profound local anesthesia upon emergence from anesthesia may be difficult for the patient to handle and can risk iatrogenic lip, tongue, and cheek biting. Medication postoperatively should match the amount and degree of dentistry performed in combination with the difficulty of anesthesia.

## POSSIBLE COMMON SIDE EFFECTS

- Nausea—can be addressed with intravenous medications and good postoperative instructions. Narcotic prescriptions are minimized when procedures are minimal or the level of understanding is limited with the patient.
- Aspiration—occasionally foreign objects or fluid can get past the airway barrier and into the lung. A foreign solid object may need to be surgically retrieved and fluid in the lung may need to be treated with oral antibiotic. A chest x-ray will help to determine the course of treatment.
- Fever—patients under anesthesia can develop fever from surgery usually from bacteremia or aspiration. The common treatment is antibiotics either intravenously or orally.

## ADDITIONAL CONCERNS

There is a growing use of the class of medication bisphosphonates. Bisphosphonates originally used to treat cancer patients have found their way into treating osteoporosis. There are two routes for delivery of bisphosphonate; the first is intravenous and the second is oral. The intravenous route has a greater risk for a condition called bone-related osteonecrosis of the jaw (BRONJ). BRONJ affects bone turnover rate and can inhibit successful healing, thus leaving exposed bone after oral surgery for a prolonged period of time.

## FINAL THOUGHTS

The beginning of this chapter posed the question as to when general anesthesia is necessary. The answer should be derived from the consideration of the mentioned medical and dental risks and benefits as described in this chapter. The final decision should be made based on input from all parties involved, including the primary care physician. The treatment plan and dental care should be predictable and maintainable by the patient or caregiver. Also, the plan should have a determined goal for oral health prevention with follow-up visits.

Hospital dentistry can be a very efficient option for patients who are medically or emotionally compromised. The availability of hospital dentistry is limited in most areas and costs can be high. General anesthesia should be the option when the other options have been considered or attempted and found to be ineffective or unsafe. Prevention with an emphasis on caries risk assessment, periodontal therapy, and remineralization strategies can help lessen the need for hospital dentistry and premature tooth loss.

# REFERENCES

Featherstone JD. (2004). The caries balance: The basis for caries management by risk assessment. *Oral Health & Preventive Dentistry* 2 (Suppl 1):259–264.

Ferguson FS, Cinotti D. (2009). Home oral health practice: The foundation for desensitization and dental care for special needs. *Dental Clinics of North America* 53:375–387, xi.

Garcia-Godoy F, Hicks MJ. (2008). Maintaining the integrity of the enamel surface: The role of dental biofilm, saliva and preventive agents in enamel demineralization and remineralization. *Journal of the American Dental Association* 139(Suppl):25S–34S.

Mallampati SR, Gatt SP, Gugino LD, et al. (1985). A clinical sign to predict difficult intubation: A prospective study. *Canadian Anaesthesiologists' Society Journal* 32:429–434.

Messieha Z. (2009). Risks of general anesthesia for the special needs dental patient. *Special Care in Dentistry* 29:21–25; quiz 67–68.

Nuckton TJ, Glidden DV, Browner WS, Claman DM. (2006). Physiological examination: Mallampati score as an independent predictor of obstructive sleep apnea. *Sleep* 29(7):903–908.

Perrott DH. (2008). Anesthesia outside the operating room in the office-based setting. *Current Opinion in Anesthesiology* 21:480–485.

Slots J. (2002). Selection of antimicrobial agents in periodontal therapy. *Journal of Periodontal Research* 37:389–398.

Waldman HB, Perlman SP, Wong A. (2008). Providing dental care for the patient with autism. *CDA Journal* 35(9):663–670.

Waldman HB, Rader R, Wong A, Perlman SP. (2009). Comorbidities and secondary conditions. *Exceptional Parent* 39(12). Available at: www.eparent.com

Weintraub JA, Ramoso-Gomez F, Jue B, Shain S, Hoover CI, Featherstone JD, Gansky SA. (2006). Fluoride varnish efficacy in preventing early childhood caries. *Journal of Dental Research* 85(2):172–176.

Wong A. (2009). Treatment planning in operating room for adult oral rehabilitation. *Dental Clinics of North America* 53:255–267.

———. (2010). *Access to Care for Special Health Care Needs Patients: Preparing the Profession for the Growing Need in Northern California*. EdD dissertation, University of the Pacific.

# 12

# Practice management tips

## David Albert Tesini, DMD, MS, FDS RCSEd

## OVERVIEW

The provision of dental services and development of a treatment philosophy must integrate into a broader network of cross-disciplinary services for patients with developmental disabilities (PWDD). These networks are constantly undergoing changes based on funding availability, changing philosophies, training of providers, and other socio-economic factors. Changing budgetary constraints of state and federal reimbursement programs demand that institutional and community-based programs funded by the public sector must be run effectively and efficiently to service PWDD in difficult economic times. The private practitioner must be prepared to address the deficiencies in the fee compensation that exist relative to the time commitment that an office must make to service and treat PWDD.

Integration of mid-level providers is intended to enhance the availability of dental care for underserved patient groups and the income disadvantaged population. Development of new workforce strategies coupled with coordinated community dental health efforts may help address some of the dental health disparities faced by PWDD. This chapter will present practice management tips across the spectrum of treatment environments.

The dental profession has historically shown its willingness to provide dental care to PWDD. Each member of the dental team must be prepared to

*Treating the Dental Patient with a Developmental Disorder*, First Edition.
Edited by Karen A. Raposa and Steven P. Perlman.
© 2012 John Wiley & Sons, Inc. Published 2012 by John Wiley & Sons, Inc.

## Willingness to $T_x$ ≠ Availability of Care

**Figure 12.1**    The willingness of providers to treat does not equal the availability of dental care to persons with developmental disabilities.

address the factors that create barriers to dental care for this population group. Unfortunately, the existence of these barriers means that, the *willingness of providers to treat patients with developmental disabilities does not translate into the availability of care for this population* (Figure 12.1).

## PROVIDING TREATMENT AND MANAGING THE PRACTICE WITHIN THE DIFFERENT TREATMENT ENVIRONMENTS

Defining the treatment objectives often involves modification of your treatment approach. Beyond the clinician having an understanding of the oral conditions that are present in different *diagnosis-specific disabilities* (Tesini & Fenton 1994), he or she must understand the varied financial challenges that exist when providing care in different clinical environments. Individuals with developmental disabilities seek care based on (1) their residential environment, (2) the awareness of their health care needs, (3) the availability of the service within the community, (4) their diagnosis-specific disability and patient characteristics (i.e., medical history, behavior, disease prevalence, etc.), (5) the proximity of the service, and (6) the philosophical orientation of the caregiver (Tesini 1987).

Optimal qualities for an ideal system have been envisioned to include (Sheller 2007):

1. Patient satisfaction.
2. Family satisfaction and partnerships.
3. Family centeredness.
4. Comprehensiveness.
5. Adequate insurance for needed services.
6. Early and continuous screening.
7. Organized community services easy for families to access and transitioning into adulthood.
8. Compliance with home care recommendations on the part of caregivers and school staff.

Practitioners and other programs have repeatedly noted problems in the provision of comprehensive dental care to individuals with disabilities (Tesini 1987; Edelstein 2007; Pradham et al. 2009; Rose et al. 2010). These include (1) limitations of the physical plant, (2) complications in time scheduling, (3) behavioral problems, (4) financial limitations for private

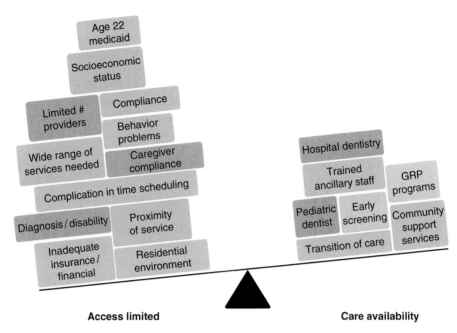

**Access limited**                                    **Care availability**

**Figure 12.2**    The fragility of the balance of access for patients with developmental disabilities.

practices to treat, (5) relatively few practitioners with adequate training, (6) capabilities of ancillary staff, and (7) guardianship and consent issues.

The *seesaw of access* defines this balance between *access* availability and *limited care* availability and functions as a class I lever in physics (Figure 12.2). The effort (force) needed to overcome the weight of the distracters (i.e., barriers) to dental care for PWDD is not in balance.

While a broad overview of community-based interventions will be covered in Chapter 13, it is important to note these options in this chapter because part of managing a private practice includes understanding the services available in the community for patients with developmental disorders. The majority of patients with disabilities receive primary services treated in four major treatment environments:

1.  The federal- or state-funded dental facility.
2.  The private dental practice.
3.  The hospital-based dental clinic.
4.  The mobile dental clinic.

Unique approaches must be found in order to overcome the barriers to care that exist for patients with developmental disabilities (Surgeon General 2000). Professional guidelines place PWDD in higher risk categories and recommend more frequent dental visits and preventive services (Crall 2007). This anticipates that the models of care and payment for care can accommodate more intensive services with greater frequency and starting at an earlier age (American Academy of Pediatric Dentistry 2010–2011).

Variation in dental care utilization within cohorts of PWDD is dependent on multiple factors including the financial burden, the source and utilization of medical care, race, insurance type, parents' education, shortage of trained providers, and the severity of the disability (Iida 2010). The extent to which dental care utilization and expenditures in PWDD differ between groups of individuals with special health care needs and the general population may truly be determined by qualitative studies of parents and providers only (Beil et al. 2009). Surely it is dependent on the successful management of the practice environment.

The Association of State & Territorial Dental Directors (ASTDD) Best Practices Project defines "best practice" as a service, function, or process that has been fine-tuned, improved, and implemented to practice "superior results." The ASTDD Best Practices Project presents state and community practice examples illustrating successful ways to implement approaches for addressing oral health issues of patients with special health care needs (Association of State & Territorial Dental Directors 2011a, 2011f).

Although the framework on which the program is based will vary depending on the population served and the program objectives, the approach to program development and management must address:

1. *Effectiveness*—does the practice "work"? Does it have the intended outcome? Does it improve, or have the potential to improve, oral health?
2. *Efficiency*—is the cost of implementing the practice, in terms of dollar cost and personnel resources, justified based on the impact?
3. *Sustainability*—does the practice have a track record of effectiveness and financial support? Is it more than a short-term project or good idea?
4. *Collaboration*—does the practice build effective partnerships among various organizations that are invested in its success, and is it integrated with broader health projects and issues?
5. *Objectives/rationale*—does the practice address Healthy People 2010 objectives or respond to the Surgeon General's Report on Oral Health? Does it build basic infrastructure and capacity for oral health programs that will persist over time?
6. *Coordination*—is the delivery of the dental care managed across all disciplines? Is there coordination and compliance with the dental health objectives? (Balzer 2007)

And we add:

7. *Integration*—have interdisciplinary partnerships within the community oriented to similar treatment goals and objectives?

The development of other initiatives such as a *mutual access program* or a *community dental facilitator project* can further allow integration of private practice and state-funded services. The mutual access model provides a "safety net" of primary generic care providers who support and rely on state-supported secondary and tertiary care that may not be available in a traditional private practice setting (Tesini 1987). Further, community facilitation at the local level can improve access to existing dental services by reducing barriers to dental care (Harrison et al. 2003).

*The following care delivery models within selected treatment environments are not intended to be interpreted as exclusive to only one treatment environment. Programs, clinics, and private practices should consider aspects of multiple models from all treatment environments. This is how the practices serving PWDD need to be developed and managed in the future.*

## Federal- and/or state-funded dental facilities

Institutional-based programs can serve both residential and community-based clients. One example of this is the Tufts Dental Facilities for Patients with Special Needs (Association of State & Territorial Dental Directors 2011g). These clinics, based at the institutions, were initially created to satisfy a legal mandate to provide care for residential clients. Later, with the realization that "institutions are in communities" (Special Care Dentistry Association 1998), community-residing clients were allowed access to comprehensive dental care. It was in this institutional dental clinic environment where most of the experienced providers were practicing (Southern Association of Institutional Dentists 2011).

The Tufts Dental Facilities model has four interwoven components:

1. *Clinical care*—since 1976, the Tufts Dental Facilities (TDF) have provided comprehensive oral health care to developmentally disabled individuals in Massachusetts. The result of a contractual partnership between the Tufts University School of Dental Medicine and the state's Department of Mental Retardation and Department of Public Health, TDF serves more than fifteen thousand patients at eight clinics throughout the state. This is the largest nationally recognized program of its kind. The program also maintains arrangements with five hospitals to address the needs of patients who require IV sedation or general anesthesia for treatment. Focused on the dental health needs of individuals with disabilities such as mental retardation, autism, blindness, and Down syndrome, the Tufts Dental Facilities draw on the support of university, community, government, hospital, and private health care resources to fill an important health care gap for this population.

2. *Community dental hygiene*—serving patients in nearly two hundred locations, the TDF Special Needs Community Dental Health Program delivers on-site dental health services to high-risk populations in schools, Head Start programs, adult day activity centers, sheltered workshops, and community residences. Nine dental hygienists travel throughout the state with portable dental equipment, providing oral health education, screening, dental cleaning, and dental sealant and fluoride application to Head Start students, students with special

needs, and other individuals. Hygienists also make referrals to local dentists and offer on-going case management services, providing a critical continuum of care that extends beyond twice-yearly cleanings.
3.   *Dental student training*—students are required to spend one week at one of the Tufts Dental Facilities.
4.   *Postgraduate GPR*—through the General Practice Residency Program, students spend about 40% of their time working with special needs patients. This provides important exposure to both the challenges and rewards of working with the special needs population.

As these types of programs develop, most of the clinical care for both institutionalized and non-institutionalized (or deinstitutionalized) people can be provided in more traditional community office settings. Other approaches that integrate well into this model have also been described:

- North Carolina institution-based—two institution-based dental clinics in North Carolina serve persons with disabilities who live in the community. Both programs have a common objective of providing access to dental care for persons with disabilities who live outside the institution and are unable to obtain care from community sources (Association of State & Territorial Dental Directors 2011b).
- Butler County—the Butler County Dental Care Program is a dental case management program sponsored by the Butler County Board of Mental Retardation and Developmental Disabilities in the state of Ohio. The program does not pay for dental services but rather integrates networks of providers, hospitals, professional organizations, case managers, caregivers, and guardian agencies. It combines existing resources to provide appropriate dental care in a timely manner to people with special needs (Association of State & Territorial Dental Directors 2011c).
- Operating Room Dental Practice—this hospital-based dental practice provides access to care for patients with special needs who require general anesthesia to obtain their treatment due to behavioral problems (Association of State & Territorial Dental Directors 2011d).
- A mutual access program, as previously discussed, is designed to support any generic system of oral care delivery.

All programs, institutional or community-based, must be driven to an efficiency level well beyond state and federal mandates to ensure long-term success and sustainability. Additional details on this topic can be found in Chapter 13.

## Private practice models

Private practices have not seen a financing system that has been responsive to the dental needs of persons with developmental disabilities. Private practice settings require a disciplined approach to managing dental care delivery that can integrate PWDD into the solo or group practice dynamic.

From office design (new or renovated) to efficient scheduling, every detail should be carefully reviewed for treatment success. Some private practices, whether general or specialty limited, develop a special care "niche,"and these referral sources should be fostered. Parents and caregivers should understand that these referrals are being made to improve care delivery.

One such private dental office is in California. A pediatric dentistry practice developed an approach that focuses directly on social and behavioral challenges specific to autism. The design of the office includes an acoustically isolated dental operatory and playroom. The "Poppy Room,"as it is called, is equipped with multisensory devices such as bubble tubes, image projectors, weighted blankets, and video glasses (Brennan 2011). Specific scheduling for this room is done with the busy pediatric dentistry environment of a private practice. Modifying the treatment environment may further enhance advanced behavior management techniques such as applied behavior analysis (Hernandez & Ikkanda 2011) and the D-Termined™ Program of Familiarization and Repetitive Tasking (Tesini 2010).

## Hospital-based dental clinics

Hospital-based dental services exist primarily to meet the needs of the low-income, uninsured, and other special patient populations. They are often university affiliated and serve as a community safety net, especially in providing emergency services. They can also function as general practice residency program centers.

All hospital departments are just that—*a hospital department*. It must function within and be part of the highly regulated hospital environment. Successful management is based on (National Maternal and Child Oral Health Resources Center 2005):

1. Shared partnerships among universities, hospitals, and community clinics.
2. Coalition of resources.
3. Defined target population—criteria for patient selection.
4. Defined services to be provided.
5. Bundling medical/dental procedures.
6. Efficient sedation/general anesthesia protocols (for more detailed information related to hospital dentistry, please refer to Chapter 11 in this book).

## Mobile dental clinics

The availability of comprehensive dental care to PWDD is probably most problematic in the rural environment and for those individuals unable to leave their living environment (Skinner et al. 2006). These dental delivery models may be based through either mobile vans or through "in-home dental teams." Mobile vans can allow for state-of-the-art equipment to your door. House calls define the latter, where "in-home dental teams" are more of a house-call model where basic dentistry is provided in the living environment and often even in the patient's bed. One such program, whose motto is "We make smiles happen at home," coordinates dental house calls by dentists and auxiliaries for homebound individuals (Portable Dental Services 2011).

The Truman Medical Center in conjunction with the Missouri Department of Health provides one of the best examples of accessible free dental services utilizing a 33-foot mobile dental van. Children and adults with developmental or intellectual disabilities in extreme financial distress, and who have found it impossible to receive care anywhere else, are eligible through referral by a local Elk's lodge (Truman Medical Center 2011).

In addition to the practice models presented, a "bridge" for compliance must be established. Partnerships with ever-changing community residential models must be fostered (Brooks et al. 2002). An example would be the use of joint commission standards and survey model (Tesini 1999) developed by Tufts Dental Facilities for use in community facilities whose clients access care through any of the treatment environments.

## Care transition from pediatric to adult oral care

Health care transitions for young adults with developmental disabilities out of the pediatric care environment present an additional management dilemma for the pediatric dental office after these patients turn 21. As pediatric dentists remain the primary community source of dental care for PWDD, offices must understand the rationale for the transition and have the knowledge and skills to manage the transition (Nowak et al. 2010). The dental home is a source of continuous and accessible professional dental care that starts soon after the eruption of the first primary tooth.

This becomes a practice management dilemma because only 10% of general dentists reported that they treat children with cerebral palsy, intellectual disability, or compounding medical conditions "often" or "very often" (Casamassimo et al. 2004).

Alternative dental health care providers may provide models that will increase access by cooperative agreements between public and private sectors. Dental hygienists with a focus on community health and preventive care are suggested as being the oral health professionals most prepared to address issues of access.

This model is intended to provide care to underserved children and families as part of a comprehensive community system of care managed by dentists. Perhaps alternative providers, such as dental therapists, will work collaboratively with dentists as part of the dental team to extend care to the underserved developmentally disabled populations (Miller 2005).

Support is building for community-driven solutions for addressing oral health access issues among vulnerable children and families. The Kellogg Foundation believes a multipronged approach—one that includes working with nonprofit advocacy groups to build community leadership in prevention, oral health literacy and a strong public health infrastructure—is critical to good oral health (Speirn 2009). Additional information on alternative health care provider models can be found in Chapter 13.

Together, providers of dental care to patients with developmental disabilities are part of the "support pyramid" needed to ensure comprehensive treatment and adequate access to care for this population (Figure 12.3).

Regardless of the model or the environment in which the treatment facility is based, support for dental services should be viewed as a "pyramid" of dental care providers. Historically, the management of this care has had too small a foundation to support a sustaining system of "access to care." The dental workforce has had little foundation to support the provision of clinical care through changes in patient demographics and funding resources. The availability of comprehensive clinical care and the quality of this care in the future will be dependent on developing this pyramid. Success will be dependent on coordinated inter-level support.

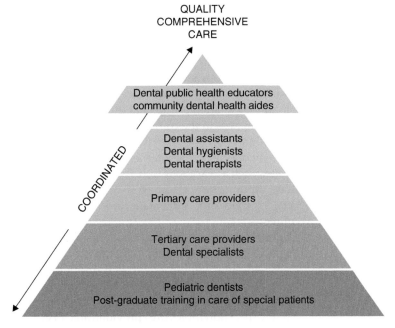

**Figure 12.3**  The support pyramid of dental providers for patients with developmental disabilities.

## MARKETING: INFORMING THE COMMUNITY THAT YOU OFFER THESE SERVICES

*Access!Access!Access!* Patients with developmental disabilities find dental care more difficult to access and purchase than other groups of individuals in "need-defined" cohorts (i.e., such as having complex medical conditions, being economically poor, being elderly, or living in alternative living environments of group homes, nursing homes, or homeless). Again, limited access is the top reason patients with developmental disabilities do not obtain dental treatment.

Over 50–90% of dentists express a willingness to treat patients W/PWDD (Kuthy et al. 2010; Iida 2010; Tsai et al. 2007; Prabhu et al. 2009). *This willingness to treat does not translate into the availability of care* (see Figure 12.1). As previously mentioned, in a survey of 1,251 general dentists, only 10% reported that they "often" or "very often" treated children with special health care needs (Casamassimo et al. 2004). The involvement of one practitioner extending care for even one patient will multiply the workforce and increase access.

This patient population has unmet dental needs for which one can become a provider—patients must know the practitioner is willing, able, and providing. Here's how to begin and refine one's approach:

- Grow it slow . . . find your niche!
- Join national and local organizations.
- Make sure the practice is listed with state dental societies and care providers (schools, parent groups, etc.).
- Develop internal efforts to create patient volume.
- Remember that one's best marketing effort is in the participation of reimbursement from the insurance plans most likely to provide coverage to this population group; that is, Medicare and Medicaid.
- Create awareness in the community to the availability of financial support through *Grotto Programs* (Grotto Program 2011).
- Social networking on the internet—start with a good Web site and link with sites such as Facebook and Twitter.
- Include your practice on Web-based provider listings such as SpecialOlympics.org, Autismlink.com, and AutismSpeaks.org.
- Volunteerism:
  1. Special Olympics—international organization that changes lives by promoting understanding, acceptance, and inclusion between people with and without intellectual disabilities through year-round sports training and athletic competition (www.specialolympics. org). Become part of the Healthy Athletes provider directory at www.specialolympics.org/providerdirectory.
  2. Best Buddies International—dedicated to providing social inclusion opportunities for people with intellectual and developmental

disabilities through their one-to-one friendship, leadership development, and supported jobs program (www.bestbuddies.org).
3. Big Brothers Big Sisters—mentoring organization in the United States where volunteers provide support and advice to youth. They nurture children and strengthen communities (www.bbbs.org).

# TRAINING YOUR STAFF FOR EFFECTIVE, EFFICIENT, AND FINANCIALLY SUSTAINABLE TREATMENT FOR PATIENTS WITH DEVELOPMENTAL DISORDERS

Since the mid-1970s, vast amounts of effort and resources have gone into improving access to care for individuals with developmental disabilities. This has resulted in a significant increase in the volume of resources available to the dental community. Although often repetitive, professional guidelines and directive protocols are available for the dental professional. This has further resulted in the availability of patient-oriented educational material and training modules that can be used by patients, parents, guardians, and direct care staff for program planning and development. Additional resources can be found in the SCDA Annual Product Guide for products useful in treating PWDD (Special Care Dentistry Association 2011c). The dental community should access this dynamic network of organizations and individuals providing care to patients with developmental disabilities.

The provision of dental care to special patient populations will not only be dentist time intensive but also staff time intensive. This awareness will directly affect the management of the clinical environment. Differences in scheduling, staff training, pre- and postappointment networking and follow-up and billing become very apparent for the practitioner integrating the care of patients with developmental disorders into the practice environment.

## Pre- and postappointment networking and follow-up

As mentioned previously in Chapters 2 and 4, directives should be reviewed with the staff. Preappointment information and patient questionnaires can be mailed or made available on your Web site. Provide help through your office as some patients and families may have difficulty in understanding the importance of this information. Together, parents and providers share knowledge and history about the patient's disability. This will allow the provider to determine the best means to deliver the care (Hernandez 2007; Tesini 2001).

## Preparing and training staff

Treatment services for patients with developmental disorders are time intensive (Tesini 2010). The reasons vary, but no one factor is greater than the need for "familiarization through repetitive tasking." Even the simplest of procedures involves slow introductions, multiple explanations, simple training steps, and repeated reinforcement. To effectively and efficiently integrate dental care of PWDD into your treatment environment, the staff must be trained, and they must accept this responsibility.

Three basic concepts can direct your staff's approach to incorporating PWDD into your practice:

1. *Behavior*—"Get into their world."
2. *Treatment planning*—"Cooperation and oral hygiene preclude treatment, but having a developmental disability does not." Individuals with developmental disabilities can receive comprehensive dental treatment . . . cooperation and oral hygiene may be limiting factors in receiving care, but having a disability is not.
3. *Financial*—"Networking, networking, networking."

*All* staff should be trained . . . but you will notice that only some staff will actually "get it." Staff must be trained to gather all the information about the patient (medical history, preappointment form, social history, etc.) and then use that information on the patient to "get into their world." Proper voice, tone, rhythm, or timing to engage both the patient and parent along with learning the right touching, holding, or stabilizing pressure are critical to effectively using behavior guidance techniques. Although most nonpharmacological techniques are based initially on familiarization, your staff should be trained to understand, and then master, the components of a successful program.

# THE D-TERMINED™ PROGRAM OF FAMILIARIZATION AND REPETITIVE TASKING

The D-Termined™ Program is based in applied behavior analysis theory and uses the "familiarization through repetitive tasking" philosophy (Hernandez & Ikkanda 2011). The D-Termined™ Program encourages us to understand that the most important factor in being successful is to be DETERMINED.

There are *three repetition factors* that are the keys to success. You must repeat these verbal commands used over and over when you use the D-Termined™ Program to guide the behavior:

1. For *eye contact*—"Look at me . . . look at me."
2. For *positional modeling*—"Put your feet out straight and hands on your tummy . . . feet out straight, hands on your tummy."

3. For a *counting framework*—verbal—"1, 2, 3, 4, 5, 6, 7, 8, 9, 10"—and/or visual; you can also use visual picture stories or counting charts.

These objectives should be reviewed with the staff and discussed with the parent. The parent will most likely recognize this approach and thank you for recognizing it as well.

With the use of these repetition commands, you can now plan the five major components of the D-Termined™ Program. Notice that they all begin with the letter D:

1. Divide the skill into small components.
   *Each step becomes a separate objective instead of a means to an end.*
   Coming into the operatory, sitting in the chair, putting the chair back, sitting in the chair with feet out straight and hands on tummy. Count finger, count fingers, count tooth, count four upper front teeth, count teeth . . . etc. A total of twenty steps are identified in dividing the tasks needed for a classic "first" visit.
2. Demonstrate the skill.
   *Positional modeling.*
   Positional modeling means that you take a skill, such as "legs out straight," and you actually put the patient's legs out straight and then support that position for a 10-second count. Follow immediately after every 10 count with praise. Continue with "hands on your tummy," meaning position the hands on the tummy and support that position with a 10-second count, followed immediately with praise . . . and so on for all of the twenty steps.
3. Drill the skill.
   *Schedule a series of five to six repetitive visits 1 week apart*
   Use the task list to divide up the tasks and skills until all are mastered and customize to each patient.
4. Delight in the repetition.
   *Everyone in the operatory remains happy, upbeat, and determined to keep trying.*
5. Delegate the patient to your trained auxiliary.
   *A trained dental auxiliary (assistant or hygienist) will start each visit and move the procedure along the step progression.*
   Later, the dentist comes into the operatory and starts at the beginning; from putting the chair back down and progressing to the point on the task list that is the objective for the day. The bulk of the repetitive tasking must be done by the auxiliary or it will become an income drain on the office regardless of the model in which care is delivered. Behavior guidance techniques MUST NOT BE DENTIST TIME INTENSIVE.

Practice with the parents or the teacher between visits is very helpful. Send them home with a disposable mirror, saliva ejector, and fluoride trays. The purpose of using the trays is to acquire the skill to tolerate tastes, impression trays, and various other materials in the mouth. Every effort should be used to help the patient tolerate fluoride trays, as it is for desensitization in preparation for impressions, mouthguards, radiographs, orthodontic retainers and appliances, and other advanced dental treatment procedures.

Morning huddles, staff meetings, and "lunch and learns," either within your office or with other like-minded offices, can increase your staff's efficiency in managing challenging behaviors. Of course, the selection of the right staff person with the proper motivation can best be effected by one-on-one training. Simple "train the trainer" programs can be integrated into any treatment environment, with your office staff training both parents and other caregivers in daily oral care principles (Nicolaci & Tesini 1982; Glassman & Miller 1998, 2006; Mabry & Mosca 2006; Special Care Dentistry Association 2011a). Other useful resources and helpful information for professional staff is readily available (Special Care Dentistry Association 2011b; International Association of Oral Health and Disability 2011; Healthy Athletes:Special Smiles 2011; Special Olympics 2011).

## Appointment scheduling considerations to meet the needs of both patients and staff

Daily routines of families with PWDD may not be easily understood by dental providers who may not have prior experience with the needs of these individuals. This accommodation needs to be balanced with the need of the dental practice to maintain a profitable financial management outcome. Scheduling of appointments must surely be viewed as a partnership between the family and the dental office. More frequent recall intervals place even greater demands to accommodate both patients and practices (Maurer et al. 1996).

# FINANCIAL REIMBURSEMENT CONSIDERATIONS FOR PRIVATE PRACTITIONERS

Unlike any other area of specialty service in dentistry, the provision of dental care to patients with developmental disabilities presents a number of challenges in how to balance the costs of providing the care. These costs often provide a financial disincentive for practitioners who otherwise are willing and able to treat. These overhead challenges include more stringent regulatory requirements, litigious attitudes, administrative cost for filing of specially coded and narrative claims, integrating of electronic medical records, and so forth. It often becomes a challenge to develop the right case mix to provide balance to fee-for-service reimbursement from so many different sources.

The private practitioner should view the financial challenge of often lower reimbursement rates per chair time for treatment of individuals with disabilities as dollar cost averaging in the financial world. In much the same way as public and private colleges and universities set and control tuition costs, so too must private practitioners be concerned with the financial implications of providing dental care to any population where reimbursement sources may pay only a percentage of the usual and customary fee. These write-offs often provide a financial disincentive that distorts the translation of dentists' willingness to treat into real access to care. Practitioners often pay closest attention to these financial issues during periods of difficult economic times and decreasing profitability. This decreasing profitability is most often due to factors *unrelated* to integrating care for special patient populations. Extrapolated from the previously discussed tuition discounting model, the following factors should be attended to for practice management success:

1. Office overhead.
2. Chair time ratios.
3. Discounted fee scale.
4. Number of patients with disabilities seen per day.
5. Business of schedule.
6. Compliance with appointments as scheduled.

The impact of the Americans with Disabilities Act has perhaps done more to enhance the availability of care than any other single factor (Americans with Disabilities Act of 1990–2011). The Internal Revenue Code has three disability-related provisions of particular interest to businesses as well as people with disabilities. Of these particularly, the tax code allows credits providing financial relief to those practices that make their offices more accessible to special needs individuals (Internal Revenue Code 2011).

Future advocacy efforts by national dental organizations should push for expansion of federal and state tax credits that might provide the necessary incentive to balance monetary shortcomings that exist when providers accept the social obligation to care for population groups that require extra time, coordination, and enhanced clinical skills.

Careful attention to overhead and development of innovative ways to manage patient care can often make for both a professionally and financially rewarding experience.

## Effective use of medical and dental billing codes and the pretreatment estimate

Writing narratives for pretreatment estimates should include:

1. A short statement of patient diagnosis.
2. Dental diagnosis.

3. Treatment needs.
4. Treatment time.
5. Requested fee.

Support your request with documentation and cross-discipline correspondence with other primary care and specialty service providers.

Dentists and patients should realize that the provision of benefits under dental insurance plans is *contract-driven*. Insurance, particularly in this population group, will determine the treatment provided. Sophisticated software has replaced much of the need for dentist consultant review. Parents and caregiver advocates must be made aware that they must be partners in securing a positive outcome on any pretreatment request.

## Billing for shorter and more frequent appointments

A New Mexico Special Needs Dental Procedure Code Program allows dentists who have completed a defined training program to submit an "encounter fee" code (SNC) for reimbursement in addition to other billable services (Association of State & Territorial Dental Directors 2011). This approach may not be applicable to other states, as it is piggybacked onto a foundation of Medicaid benefits for adults.

## Services that are donated in response to unmet needs

Many patients with developmental disabilities are covered under public health programs such as Medicaid, Medicare, and the State Children's Health Insurance Program (SCHIP). These programs, mandated to provide basic preventive and restorative care, are chronically underfunded and age sensitive. PWDD are often included in studies of oral health of underserved populations (Tiller et al. 2001; Dolan et al. 2005). Services by dental providers that have not been reimbursed by state or federal programs, dental insurance companies, or out-of-pocket payers have been estimated to exceed $1.6 billion (Manski et al. 1999). The Demographics and distribution of these services vary.

Tens of thousands of dentists provide free dental care to hundreds of thousands of disadvantaged and disabled people each year through volunteer programs, such as the ADA "Give Kids a Smile" (www.givekidsasmile. org), "Dental Lifeline Network" (www.nfdh.org) and "Missions of Mercy" (www.acdfmom.org) (American Dental Association 2010). The Dental Lifeline Network is a charitable affiliate of the ADA and coordinates the services of thousands of volunteer dentists and laboratories nationwide to provide comprehensive dental care to vulnerable patients in need of dental care.

# SUMMARY

To integrate PWDD into the clinical dental practice environment the clinician/manager must develop an efficient and effective management system. How will the dental community participate in providing care to these populations? Were they adequately trained in caring for the patient with special needs? Will the providers' commitment be limited to the private practice environment or can they also be involved in academic, community, or institutionally based clinics? Do they have a desire to become a director and shape models of care delivery? Will treatment of patients in the special patient arena become career defining for some gifted providers?

From these practice management tips, dental providers can develop their own delivery models to integrate PWDD, provide access to an underserved population, and grow their careers.

# REFERENCES

American Academy of Pediatric Dentistry. (2010–2011). Guideline on dental management of dental patients with special health care needs. *Journal of Pediatric Dentistry* 32(6):132–136.

American Dental Association. Donated care. http://www.ada.org/2389.aspx, accessed November 15, 2010.

Americans with Disabilities Act of 1990. (2011). Americans with Disabilities Act of 1990 [ADA], including changes made by the ADA Amendments Act of 2008 (P.L. 110-325). Accessed February 1, 2011, from http://www.ada.gov/pubs/adastatute08.pdf.

Association of State & Territorial Dental Directors. (2011a). Accessed January 30, 2011, from http://www.astdd.org/special-health-care-needs-introduction/.

———. (2011b). Accessed January 30, 2011, from http://www.astdd.org/best-practices/pdf/DES36003NCspecial needsinstitutionservices.pdf.

———. (2011c). Accessed January 30, 2011, from http://www.astdd.org/best-practices/pdf/DES38006OHspecial needscasemanagement.pdf.

———. (2011d). Accessed January 30, 2011, from http://www.astdd.org/best-practices/pdf/DES38007OHspecial needsoperatingroom.pdf.

———. (2011e). Accessed January 30, 2011, from http://www.astdd.org/state-activities-descriptive-summaries/ ?id=190.

———. (2011f). Accessed January 30, 2011, from http://www.astdd.org/special-health-care-needs/bestpracticeapproach.

———. (2011g). Accessed January 30, 2011, from http://www.astdd.org/best-practices/pdf/DES24005MAspecial needstuftsfacilities.pdf.

Balzer J. (2007). Improving systems of care for people with special needs: The ASTDD Best Practices Project. *Journal of Pediatric Dentistry* 29(2):123–128.

Beil H, Mayer M, Rozier G. (2009). Dental care utilization and expenditures in children with special health care needs. *Journal of the American Dental Association* 140(9):1147–1155.

Brennan L, Price S. (2011). Accessed January 30, 2011, from http://oakparkden tistryforchildren.com/special_needs_patients.html.

Brooks C, et al. (2002). Program evaluation of mobile dental services for children with special health care needs. *Special Care Dentistry* 22(4):156–160.

Casamassimo PS, Seale NS, Ruehs K. (2004). General dentists' perceptions of educational and treatment issues affecting access to care for children with special health care needs. *Journal of Dental Education* 68(1):23–28.

Crall JJ. (2007). Improving oral health for individuals with special health care needs. *Journal of Pediatric Dentistry* 29(2):98–104.

Dolan TA, Atchison K, Huynh TN. (2005). Access to dental care among older adults in the Unites States. *Journal of Dental Education* 69(9):961–974.

Edelstein BL. (2007). Conceptual frameworks for understanding system capacity in the care of people with special health care needs (conference paper). *Journal of Pediatric Dentistry* 29(2):108–116.

Glassman P, Miller CE. (1998). Improving oral health for people with special needs through community based dental care delivery systems. *Journal of the California Dental Association* 26(5):404–409.

———. (2006). Effect of preventive dentistry training programs for caregivers in community facilities on caregiver and client behavior and client oral hygiene. *New York State Dental Journal* 72(2):38–46.

Grotto Program. (2011). Accessed January 30, 2011, from http://www.masonin info.com/dentistry.htm.

Harrison RL, Li J, Pearce K, et al. (2003). The Community Dental Facilitator Project: Reducing barriers to dental care. *Journal of Public Health Dentistry* 63(3):126–128.

Healthy Athletes:Special Smiles. (2011). Accessed February 1, 2011, from http:// media.specialolympics.org/soi/files/healthy-athletes/Special%20_Smiles_ Good_Oral_Health_Guide.pdf.

Hernandez P, Ikkanda Z. (2011). Applied behavior analysis: Behavior management of children with autism spectrum disorders in dental environments. *Journal of the American Dental Association* 142:281–287.

Hernandez PJ. (2007). Perspectives of a parent and a provider for children with special health care needs. *Journal of Pediatric Dentistry* 29(2):105–107.

Iida H, Lewis C, Zhou C, et al. (2010). Dental care needs, use and expenditures among U.S. children with and without special health care needs. *Journal of the American Dental Association* 141(1):79–88.

Internal Revenue Code. (2011). Disabled Access Tax Credit (Title 26, Section 44); Tax Deduction to Remove Architectural and Transportation Barriers to People with Disabilities and Elderly Individuals (Title 26, Section 190); Targeted Jobs Tax Credit (Title 26, Section 51). Accessed February 1, 2011, from http://www.irs.gov/businessess/small/article/0,,id=185704,00.html.

International Association of Oral Health and Disability. (2011). Accessed February 1, 2011, from http://www.iadh.org/links/.

Kuthy RA, McQuistan MR, et al. (2010). Dental students' perceived comfort and willingness to treat underserved populations: Surveys prior to and immediately after extramural experiences. *Journal of Special Care Dentistry* 30(6):242–249.

Mabry CC, Mosca NG. (2006). Interprofessional educational partnerships in school health for children with special oral health needs. *Journal of Dental Education* 70(8):844–850.

Manski RJ, Moeller JF, Maas WR. (1999). Dental services: Use, expenditures and sources of payment. *Journal of the American Dental Association* 130(4): 500–508.

Maurer SM, Boggs AM, Mourino AP, et al. (1996). Recall intervals: Effect on treatment needs of the handicapped patient; a retrospective study. *Journal of Clinical Pediatric Dentistry* 20(2):123–126.

Miller CE. (2005). Access to care for people with special needs: Role of alternative providers and practice settings. *Journal of the California Dental Association* 33(9):715–721.

National Maternal and Child Oral Health Resources Center. (2005). Oral health for children and adolescents with special health care needs: Challenges and opportunities. Available at: http://www.mchoralhealth.org/PDFs/SHCNfactsheet.pdf.

Nicolaci AB, Tesini D. (1982). Improvement in the oral hygiene of institutionalized mentally retarded individuals through training of direct care staff: A longitudinal study. *Journal of Special Care Dentistry* 2(5):217–221.

Nowak AJ, Casamassimo PS, Slaxton RL. (2010). Facilitating the transition of patients with special health care needs from pediatric to adult oral health care. *Journal of the American Dental Association* 141(11):1351–1356.

Portable Dental Services. (2011). Accessed January 30, 2011, from http://www.portabledentalservices.com.

Prabhu NT, Nunn JH, Evans DJ, et al. (2009). Access to dental care: Parents' and caregivers' views on dental treatment services for people with disabilities. *Special Care in Dentistry* 30:35–45.

Pradham A, Slade GD, Spencer AJ. (2009). Access to dental care among adults with physical and mental disabilities: Residence factors. *Australian Dental Journal* 54(3):204–211.

Rose RA, Parish SL, Yoo J, et al. (2010). Suppression of racial disparities for children with special health care needs among families receiving Medicaid. *Social Science & Medicine* 70(9):1263–1270.

Sheller B. (2007). Systems Issues Workshop report (conference paper). *Journal of Pediatric Dentistry* 29(2):150–152.

Skinner AC, Slifkin RT, Mayer ML. (2006). The effect of rural residence on dental unmet need for children with special health care needs. *Journal of Rural Health* 22(1):36–42.

Southern Association of Institutional Dentists. (2011). Accessed January 30, 2011, from http://www.saiddent.org.

Special Care Dentistry Association. (1998). A position paper from the Academy of Dentistry for persons with disabilities: "Preservation of quality oral health services for people with developmental disabilities." *Special Care Dentistry* 18(5):180–183.

———. (2011a). Special care: An oral health professional's guide to serving young children with special health care needs. Accessed February 1, 2011, from http://www.mchoralhealth.org/specialcare/index.htm.

———. (2011b). Accessed February 1, 2011, from http://www.scdonline.org/displaycommon.cfm?an=1&subarticlebr=81.

———. (2011c). Special Care Dentistry Association Annual Product Guide. Accessed January 30, 2011, from http://www.scdonline.org/associations/2865/files/SDCNov-Dec07-ProdGuide.pdf.

Special Olympics. (2011). Accessed February 1, 2011, from http://resources.specialolympics.org/sections/healthy_althletes_resources.aspx.

Speirn SK. (2009). Strengthening oral care is the key part of health reform. Accessed January 30, 2011, from http://www.wkkf.org/news/Articles/2009/11/Strengthening-Oral-Health-Care-is-Key-Part-of-Health-Reform.aspx.

Surgeon General. (2000). Oral health in America: A report of the Surgeon General. Available at: http://www.surgeongeneral.gov/library/oralhealth/.

Tesini D. (1987). Providing dental services for citizens with handicaps: A prototype community program. *Journal of Mental Retardation* 25(4):219–222.

———. (1999). Oral health care for community residences: Improving oral health through performance measurement. Available at: http://specializedcare.com/shop/pc/viewcontent.asp?idpage=6.

———. (2001). Finding your care in the parking lot: The role of parents and direct support professionals in providing attention to oral health care needs of the child with special needs. *Exceptional Parent Magazine*, October, pp. 89 ff.

———. (2010). The D-Termined™ Program of Familiarization and Repetitive Tasking. *Practical Reviews in Pediatric Dentistry* 24(4)30. (Audio presentation August 30, 2010.)

Tesini DA, Fenton S. (1994). Oral health needs of persons with physical or mental disabilities. *Dental Clinics of North America* 38(3):483–498.

Tiller S, Wilson KI, Gallagher JE. (2001). Oral health status and dental service use of adults with learning disabilities living in residential institutions and in the community. *Community Dental Health* 18(3):167–171.

Truman Medical Center. (2011). Accessed January 30, 2011, from http://www.trumed.org/trumed/lw/lw_medical_care/lw_health_services/lw_elks_dental_van.aspx.

Tsai WC, et al. (2007). Changes and factors associated with dentists' willingness to treat patients with severe disabilities. *Health Policy* 83(2):363–374.

# 13

# Improving oral health through community-based interventions

## Paul Glassman, DDS, MA, MBA

## INTRODUCTION

Analysis of the factors that allow people to live long, healthy lives reveals that the most important factor is behaviors that can be controlled by the individual (McGinnis & Foege 1993; McGinnis et al. 2002). In fact, the factors that lead to long, healthy lives can be grouped roughly as follows:

- 40%—individual behaviors. Examples include reduction or elimination of the use of tobacco, moderate consumption of alcohol, and in the case of oral health, plaque removal and use of fluoride and other products that alter the oral environment.
- 30%—genetics. At present we can only mitigate a small number of the genetic factors that cause disability, illness, and early death, although there are many treatments available for the results of our genetic makeup and new discoveries being made in this area at a dramatic rate.
- 20%—environment and public health measures. These include steps to reduce pollution, overcrowding, and stress, and public health measures such as sanitation, immunization, and fluoridation of the drinking water.
- 10%—procedures performed by health care professionals.

The last bullet point should get our attention. We put most of our health care resources in the United States into procedures performed by heath care professionals, and yet they account for such a small portion of the factors that lead to long, healthy lives.

*Treating the Dental Patient with a Developmental Disorder*, First Edition.
Edited by Karen A. Raposa and Steven P. Perlman.
© 2012 John Wiley & Sons, Inc. Published 2012 by John Wiley & Sons, Inc.

Although the data described above come from an analysis of general health conditions, it seems likely that roughly the same proportions would hold for oral health. If this is the case, then it follows that to keep a population of people having good oral health requires more emphasis on influencing behaviors and less on relying on oral health professionals to repair the ravages of disease after they have occurred. This is especially true when considering people with disabilities, where, in general, treatment of existing disease is more complex and at times more costly than with other segments of the population (Glassman & Miller 2009).

Another issue to consider is the reach of office-based oral health care. Over 30% of the population does not take advantage of the traditional office-based dental delivery system (ADA 2006). This proportion is even higher in people with low income and those with physical and medical disabilities. Since disability is often associated with low income, and people with disabilities may be more difficult to treat, they are among the least likely to receive oral health care in traditional office-based delivery systems and have been identified as being among the populations with the greatest oral health disparities (U.S. Bureau of the Census 1997; Stiefel 2001; U.S. Department of Health and Human Services 2000).

In addition, consider the ability of office-based practices to influence individual behaviors and emphasize prevention and early intervention. This is challenging for several reasons. First, as indicated above, people with disabilities are among the least likely to take advantage of office-based care. In addition, dental offices are intimidating for many people and are not the environment where people are the most open and ready to listen to and integrate oral health messages. Also, the economics of dental practice encourages providers to spend the majority of their time and effort on technical procedures requiring the sophisticated equipment and the highly skilled professionals found in these environments.

All of these factors lead to the conclusion that systems capable of influencing individual behaviors and emphasizing prevention and early intervention may best be developed and delivered in community settings. This chapter will describe what the author means by community-based settings and provide examples of community-based systems that have been shown to be effective in improving the oral health of people with disabilities.

# WHAT ARE COMMUNITY-BASED SETTINGS AND COMMUNITY-BASED SYSTEMS OF CARE?

As used in this chapter, the term "community-based settings" can include any location outside of a dental office environment. However, the emphasis in this chapter will be on settings where people may be grouped together to receive social, general health, or educational services. Many people with disabilities, particularly those with significant disabilities, live or spend time in group settings (Glassman & Subar 2010). Group settings can include schools, group residential facilities, long-term care facilities, and child and adult day-care settings. People with disabilities may also be seen by numerous social and health professionals in the process of receiving home-based social and general health services. All of these sites and situations present opportunities to integrate oral health activities with the activities of professionals, staff, and caregivers who interact with people with disabilities in community settings.

Community-based systems of care are delivery mechanisms that take place within the context of the services and settings just described. There are a number of common elements that may be included in oral health care that is delivered in community-based oral health systems. These include case management, community-based health education, community-based prevention procedures, community-based therapeutic interventions, and elements of the patient-centered health home (ADA 2004; Bernabei et al. 1998; DeBate et al. 2006; Park et al. 2009; Mertz & O'Neil 2002; Zittel-Palamara et al. 2005).

The patient-centered health home has been described as a system of care that provides care management over time; health promotion activities; access to technical medical services when needed; and in pediatric medical home models, there is also an emphasis on early intervention services (Beal et al. 2007). Many descriptions of medical homes or health homes describe them as taking place within the primary physician's or dentist's office (American Academy of Pediatric Dentistry 2011; National Association of State Health Policy 2009). However, there is increasing realization that the elements of a patient-centered health home can be achieved by many different structures and the primary care provider's office does not need to be the center of the entity that delivers and coordinates these services (Pacific Center for Special Care 2011).

The remainder of this chapter will describe several examples of community-based systems that can create or extend components of the patient-centered health home to people with disabilities.

# EXAMPLES OF COMMUNITY-BASED SYSTEMS OF CARE

## The dental coordinator model

There are numerous examples of systems that deliver oral health services and improve the oral health of people with disabilities in community set-tings. Almost 2 decades ago the Pacific Center for Special Care created a community-based system of care in conjunction with the California Regional Center System (Glassman & Miller 1994, 1998, 2009; Glassman et al. 1996). Regional Centers are social service agencies with long-term contracts with the California Department of Developmental Services that provide assessment, case management, and referral services for people with developmental disabilities. The center of the oral health system is an individual referred to as the "Dental Coordinator" (DC). Dental Coordinators are primarily dental hygienists who work for and sometimes in the Regional Center office in communities across California. They act as a "dental case manager." Their role includes the following activities:

- Leverage local resources—this involves determining what resources already exist in a community and facilitating communication among those resources. In many communities, there are practitioners willing to treat some people with developmental disabilities and social service agency personnel who did not know about these oral health professionals. One role of the DC is to make these individuals aware of each other.
- Develop local resources—in many communities, there is at least one critical resource in short supply or totally lacking. In some communities the DCs, with assistance and consultation from the authors, have helped set up hospital facilities and protocols and trained community dentists to work in a hospital environment. In other communities, developing local resources involves working with individual dental offices to support them in seeing people with developmental disabilities that are prescreened to be sure they are appropriate to receive care in that office.
- Screen, triage, refer, track, and manage emergency and routine dental care—in many communities the DC conducts screening clinics to identify individuals in need of dental services. Screening information collected includes dental findings, predictions about dental treatment needed, predictions about the individual's ability to cooperate for dental treatment in a dental office, and recommendations about the best setting for receiving future dental care. Individuals are then referred to appropriate treatment resources and tracked to be sure that they receive the care they need.
- Conduct individual and group prevention programs—the DC identifies opportunities to provide oral health prevention education. In some cases this is provided in individual settings and sometimes in groups. In a number of communities, the DC is involved in ensuring that an individual who had dental treatment in a hospital under general anesthesia is involved in an intensive prevention program to reduce the need for further treatment in that environment. The DCs create and help caregivers implement individual oral health prevention plans for people with developmental disabilities.
- Integrate oral health considerations into agency systems—a critical component of the system and an important focus of the DC is to find ways to integrate oral health into activities in place in social service and general health systems. This involves including oral health information in intake processes; integrating oral health considerations in individual and program planning activities; and enlisting social and general health professionals in identifying the risk for oral disease and providing oral health prevention information.

In one 3-year demonstration of this model there was significant improvement in the oral health of the population being served (Glassman & Miller 2009). This system has spread to include the majority of the Regional Center Systems in California.

## Integration of oral health into social service and general health systems

Another approach to improving the oral health of people with developmental disabilities in community settings is to train and support social service and general health professionals to make assessments of oral health risk and to deliver oral health services.

The Pacific Center for Special Care at the University of the Pacific School of Dentistry has developed a program to train social workers and nurses who perform assessment and referral services for families enrolled in the California Regional Center's Early Start program (California Department of Developmental Services 2011). This program serves families of young children at risk of having a developmental disability. Because the program serves mainly low-income and minority and diverse families it is very difficult to make referrals to dental offices for evaluation and education.

Nurses and social workers who act as Infant Service Coordinators in the Early Start System receive training on the causes and prevention of early childhood caries. They are provided a questionnaire that asks parents questions about concerns, previous oral health care, and dietary and prevention habits. They are also taught to look for white spot lesions or holes in the teeth. Based on the answers to these questions, the children in this program are classified as being at low, medium, or high risk for developing dental caries. For those at low and medium risk, the nurse or social worker is able to provide education and leave language-appropriate educational materials with the family. The nurse or social worker also applies a fluoride varnish. For those at higher risk or who require other interventions, the nurse or social worker is able to use the services of a Dental Coordinator employed by the social service agency for further education or help with referral to a dental office. Using this system, only 25% of families need referral to a dental office for further guidance or treatment. Reducing the number of referrals needed makes it much more likely that any single referral will be successful.

Similar approaches have been used to train physicians to identify children at risk for oral disease and perform appropriate interventions (Maryland's Mouths Matter 2011). In California a law took effect January 1, 2010, that allows anyone to apply fluoride varnish to the teeth of a person being served in a public health setting or program that is created or administered by a state or local governmental entity if the application is in accordance with a prescription and protocol issued and established by a physician or dentist (California Health and Safety Code 2011).

These efforts must be expanded to ensure that general health, social service, and education professionals are aware of and assess the risk for oral disease and are trained to provide appropriate intervention.

## The virtual dental home

One new model of care for underserved populations, including people with developmental disabilities, is being demonstrated in California and is called the Virtual Dental Home (VDH) (Pacific Center for Special Care 2011). The VDH system is a community-based oral health delivery system in which people receive preventive and simple therapeutic services in community settings where they live or receive educational, social, or general health services. It utilizes the latest technology to link practitioners in the community with dentists at remote office sites. The goal is to demonstrate that allied dental professionals can keep people healthy in community settings by providing education, preventive care, interim therapeutic restorations triage, and case management. Where more complex dental treatment is needed, the VDH system connects patients with dentists in the area.

This system promotes collaboration between dentists in dental offices and these community-based allied dental professionals. Most importantly, it brings much-needed services to individuals who might otherwise receive no care.

This model relies on the advanced training and community-based practice of a group of allied oral health professionals. They collaborate with a dentist to a full system of care. Technology helps bridge the geographic gap between the community provider and the dentist.

Equipped with portable imaging equipment and an internet-based dental record system, allied dental professionals collect electronic dental records such as x-rays, photographs, charts of dental findings, and dental and medical histories, and upload the information to a secure Web site where they are reviewed by a collaborating dentist. The dentist reviews the patient's information and creates a tentative dental treatment plan. The allied dental professional then carries out the aspects of the treatment plan that can be conducted in the community setting. These services include:

- Health promotion and prevention education.
- Dental disease risk assessment.
- Preventive procedures such as application of fluoride varnish, dental sealants, and, for dental hygienists, dental prophylaxis and periodontal scaling.
- Placing carious teeth in a holding pattern using interim therapeutic restorations (ITRs) to stabilize patients until they can be seen by a dentist for definitive care.
- Tracking and supporting the individual's need for and compliance with recommendations for additional and follow-up dental services.

The allied dental professionals refer patients to dental offices for procedures that require the skills of a dentist. When such visits occur, the patient arrives with a diagnosis and treatment plan already determined, preventive practices in place, and preventive procedures having been performed. The patient is likely to receive a successful first visit with the dentist and require fewer visits as the patient's dental records and images have already been reviewed. In some cases the dentist may come to the community site and use portable equipment to provide restorations or other services that only a dentist can provide. In either case, the majority of patient interactions and efforts to keep people healthy are performed by the allied dental professionals in the community setting, thus creating a true community-based dental home.

While the VDH system is being successfully demonstrated in pilot sites across California, it will require regulatory and reimbursement reform in most states to be able to spread. However, many states could develop variations of this model that could bring much-needed care to people with developmental disabilities.

## CONCLUSION

This chapter is based on the assertion that developing and deploying community-based systems of care is a critical and often missing element in current dental care delivery systems. In some situations there are clear and readily achievable steps that can be taken to extend dental practices into the community; add oral health activities to existing social, educational, or general health systems; or develop partnerships between oral health and social service, educational, or general health systems. In other cases these partnerships are not so readily available and creativity is required.

It is also clear that comprehensive oral health systems for people with disabilities will not become widespread without policy changes and regulatory and reimbursement reforms directed at removing barriers to and providing support for these systems. It is hoped that oral health professionals and others concerned about improving and maintaining oral health for people with disabilities will realize the importance of establishing and supporting these important systems of care.

## REFERENCES

American Academy of Pediatric Dentistry. (2011). Policy on the dental home. Revised 2004; adopted 2011.

American Dental Association (ADA). (2004). State and community models for improving access to dental care for the underserved—a white paper.

————. (2006). Review of existing data on the adequacy of the current workforce, need for care, and the impact of expanded duties on access to care. ADA House of Delegates Resolution 3, Appendix 2.

Beal AC, Dory MM, Hernandez SE, et al. (2007). Closing the divide: How medical homes promote equity in health care: Results from the Commonwealth Fund 2006 Health Care Quality Survey. The Commonwealth Club.

Bernabei R, Landi F, Gambassi G, et al. (1998). Randomized trial of impact of model of integrated care and case management for older people living in the community. *British Medical Journal* 316(7141):1348–1351.

California Department of Developmental Services. (2011). Early Start home page. http://www.adds.ca.gov/earlystart/ Accessed April 20, 2011, from www.dds.ca.gov/EarlyStart/Home.cfm

California Health and Safety Code. (2011). Section 104830.

DeBate RD, Plichta SB, Tedesco LA, Kerschbaum WE. (2006). Integration of oral health care and mental health services: Dental hygienists' readiness and capacity for secondary prevention of eating disorders. *Journal of Behavioral Health Services & Research* 33(1):113–125.

Glassman P, Miller C. (1994). A dental school's role in developing a community based dental care delivery system for persons with developmental disabilities. *Journal of Dental Education* 58(2):133.

————. (1998). Improving oral health for people with special needs through community-based dental care delivery Systems. *CDA Journal* 26(5):404–409.

————. (2009). Social supports and prevention strategies as adjuncts and alternatives to sedation and anesthesia for people with special needs. *Special Care in Dentistry* 29(1):31–38.

Glassman P, Miller C, Lechowick J. (1996). A dental school's role in developing a rural, community-based dental care delivery system for individuals with developmental disabilities. *Special Care in Dentistry* 29 16(5):188–193.

Glassman P, Subar P. (2010). Creating and maintaining oral health for dependent people in institutional settings. *Journal of Public Health Dentistry* 70:S40–S48.

Maryland's Mouths Matter. (2011). Fluoride varnish and oral health screening program for kids—training for EPSDT medical providers in Maryland. http://www.ohmdkids.org/flvarnish/Index.html Accessed April 20, 2011, from www.mchoralhealth.org/flvarnish/index.html.

McGinnis JM, Foege WH. (1993). Actual causes of death in the United States. *Journal of the American Medical Association* 270(18):2207–2212.

McGinnis JM, Williams-Russo P, Knickman JR. (2002). The case for more active policy attention to health promotion. *Health Affairs* 21(2):78–93.

Mertz E, O'Neil E. (2002). The growing challenge Of providing oral health care services to all Americans. *Health Affairs* 21(5):65–77.

National Association of State Health Policy. (2009). Building medical homes in state Medicaid and CHIP programs.

Pacific Center for Special Care at the University of the Pacific School of Dentistry. (2011). The virtual dental home. Accessed April 1, 2011, from http://dental.pacific.edu/Community_Involvement/Pacific_Center_for_Special_Care_(PCSC)/Projects/Virtual_Dental_Home_Demonstration_Project.html.

Park EJ, Huber DL, Tahan HA. (2009). The evidence base for case management practice. *Western Journal of Nursing Research* 31(6):693–714.

Stiefel DJ. (2001). Adults with disabilities. Dental care considerations of disadvantages and special care populations: Proceedings of the conference. Held April 18–19, 2001, in Baltimore, Maryland. U.S. Department of Health and Human Services, Health Resources and Services Administration, Bureau of Health Professions, Division of Medicine and Dentistry, Division of Nursing.

U.S. Bureau of the Census. (1997). Americans with disabilities: 1994–95. Current Population Reports. P70-61. Census Brief, CENBR/97-5 Washington DC: U.S. Department of Commerce, Economics and Statistics Administration.

U.S. Department of Health and Human Services. (2000). Oral health in America: A report of the Surgeon General. Rockville, MD: U.S. Department of Health and Human Services, National Institute of Dental and Craniofacial Research, National Institutes of Health.

Zittel-Palamara K, Fabiano JA, Davis EL. (2005). Improving patient retention and access to oral health care: The CARES program. *Journal of Dental Education* 69(8):912–918.

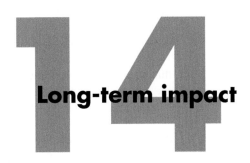

# 14

# Long-term impact

Jo Ann Simons, MSW

True story: A mother brings her two young children into the dental office for a checkup and cleaning. The older child, Jon, is a boy of 10, and he is well mannered and easygoing. He sits compliantly for the entire session. The younger child, a girl, is 6. She is antsy and can't sit still. She gags whenever the dentist comes near her mouth and she bites him. Fortunately, the dentist is wearing a guard. With great ease Jon's exam is finished. Emily, the younger girl, requires more attention and time. Her behavior does not improve much for a few more years. What is remarkable is that Jon, the young boy, the easy patient, has Down syndrome and congenital heart disease. He grows up to own a home, drive a car, graduate college, and work on a golf course. The girl, what is sometimes referred to as a *neuro-typical child* (a term I dislike), is a very difficult patient. While she eventually grows up to be a successful attorney, there was no predicting it that day in the dental office. I should know. They are both my children. The lesson here is the same one that my family tried to instill in me and that your family hopefully taught you—don't judge people by how they look on the outside. What matters most is on the inside.

If you think that you can judge your patient's behavior on how he or she looks, let me tell you—you will not be able to take a look at a patient and determine his or her attitude, behavior, or even if the individual will pay his or her bills.

I am writing this chapter so that if someone like me walks into your dental office with a child with a disability, or with an adult child with a disability, you might take a moment to see the individual and not the

*Treating the Dental Patient with a Developmental Disorder*, First Edition.
Edited by Karen A. Raposa and Steven P. Perlman.
© 2012 John Wiley & Sons, Inc. Published 2012 by John Wiley & Sons, Inc.

disability. I hope you will see a child or an adult with a disability as a patient needing your care. Because I will be looking for a competent dentist with compassion and warmth.

Those characteristics—competency, compassion, and warmth—are ones that you should be hoping you have for a successful practice. In fact, they are good characteristics for success because nobody is interested in a competent dentist with a lousy attitude.

When a child is born or diagnosed with an intellectual disability/developmental disability (ID/DD), after the shock and awe, the family begins to look for acceptance. Usually, it is family members and close friends who provide the support that is essential for the family to regain their footing and strength as they enter a world they are largely unprepared for.

I was lucky. When my son was born, I was surrounded by a supportive family and a medical team of unmatched expertise. My father actually built a virtual mountain for Jon to climb, with goals that many might have said were unrealistic. But every goal was reached: reading, writing, going away to sleep-away camp for 8 weeks every summer, breaking 100 for a round of golf, graduating high school, owning a home, having a job, having a girlfriend, and driving a car.

There are hundreds of people who can claim to be part of Jon's success and my healing. And they are proud, and should be, of their contributions to a good life.

For me, part of my healing came from a dentist. I was at the beach, many years ago, with my toddler son, who was born with Down syndrome and tetralogy of Fallot. A handsome young man approached Jon and me. At first, I thought that this young man was flirting with me (or at least I hoped). As he began to speak to me, he showed more interest in Jon than me. In fact, he made many positive and affirming comments about my beautiful baby. As our conversation continued, I learned that he was a pediatric dentist and had experience with children like my son. Ironically, 6 months earlier, I had been given his name as a dentist who was as skillful as he was kind. That day on the beach, we both found gifts; my son found a dentist and I found my dear friend Dr. Steven Perlman.

You have an opportunity right now to decide what kind of dentist you will become. Will you be inclusive of all people needing your care, or will you cherry-pick ones that look or act a certain way? It is your life and your career and soon it will be your time to decide whether to stand up and be counted or just show up.

Many families with children with ID/DDs feel different. They fight for acceptance for their children from schools, sports leagues, and even religious organizations. They do not want to have to fight for access to quality dental care. They want the same thing as you want for yourself and for your family—good care.

What kind of reputation do you want? Someone who will be recommended for both his or her competency and decency? Do you want to be known as someone to avoid if you have a child with a disability? Do you want to treat whole families? Do you want to be inclusive?

Regardless of whether you intend to be a general dentist or specialize, individuals with ID/DDs and their families are potential patients. They have the same need to have access to quality and compassionate care. While ID/DD may not have touched you personally, at least not yet, you have certainly attended school, attended religious services, or played on sports teams with persons with ID/DDs. You know that they are more alike than different from you.

In fact, as you have learned from other chapters in this book, they often have unique dental needs. They are often interesting patients.

In my son's case, he has no dental caries, which is not unusual for someone with Down syndrome. He is able to keep his wisdom teeth, a gift from his father. His teeth erupted in fairly typical fashion and came in straight and he didn't need braces. However, he did need to have a couple of teeth bonded because they ended in points. That was 18 years ago and having good-looking teeth is important for anyone, and I would say it is even more important for someone with a disability.

If only it took an apple a day to maintain health and wellness, we would all invest in apples. Families know that finding access to quality dental care for individuals with ID/DDs takes more than apples. It can sometimes feel like an endless journey. Families also face the same burden of paying for dental care as other families.

When the child becomes an adult, there can be many changes—access can become even more limited and the reimbursement system can become more difficult. Families have found that finding quality adult dental care is very challenging, and many families find themselves having to educate dental health professionals about the dental needs of their child. Families have had to make a lifetime commitment to their child's oral health, and they are only asking that you become partners in this part of their journey along with others who help care for their child. Many individuals with ID/DDs have some special considerations related to health care, and you could become an important member—along with other medical professionals—of an individual's health care team.

In thinking about writing this chapter, I wanted to learn why people want to become dentists. I learned that for many young people, besides the opportunity to be well compensated, dentistry provides a superior lifestyle compared to, let's say, medicine. On one message board, this comment resonated with me because it makes dentists the ideal professionals to work with individuals with ID/DDs:

> I think what sucked me into dentistry had to be the idea of personally being able to determine my lifestyle, and also receive an incredible amount of patient interaction. I've shadowed a bunch of places, and I must say, my experiences with the dentists I have worked with have all been quite a motivation to enter the field.

Contrary to what the public sometimes believes, these dentists are truly happy doing their work. I'd like to be like that too. The money is of course a benefit, but certainly falls short of being the reason I am pursuing dentistry. I also am a pretty detail oriented person, something I think is needed in dentistry. All in all, the interaction with people and medical aspect caught my eye initially.

Here is what I gleaned from this comment: *dentistry provides financial benefit, ability to interact with patients, appeals to people good at details, and provides for a good lifestyle.*

People with ID/DDs might give you what you are looking for in a patient.

Individuals with ID/DDs often have complex medical needs, from on-going issues related to congenital heart disease to adult issues including new physical and mental health concerns. There is the need to pay attention to detail. Our children can be expected to live longer lives and, as a result, face aging issues, including Alzheimer's disease. We need dentists who are comfortable with our children throughout their lives.

Families often spend considerable time finding the right dentist for their child. They ask around, get some recommendations, and then they might make some telephone calls and discuss their child with the office staff. Once a family finds someone who seems to be able to meet their expectations for a dentist, they might make an appointment and take their child in to see if it is a good match.

Even if you might have some hesitations in meeting the needs of a patient with an ID/DD, families are often willing to help you understand the needs of their son or daughter. Families are really the experts when it comes to caring for their child.

It is also a two-way street. Since reputation and word-of-mouth referrals are the most important marketing tools you have, paying attention to this population can help you build a practice. People with children with disabilities tell other families what to look for in a dentist. We tell families to consider the following factors:

- The doctor's experience with intellectual and developmental disabilities.
- Whether the doctor is committed to the highest quality of life for your child.
- Office hours.
- Your child's comfort level with the dentist.
- Whether the doctor respects your child and communicates with him or her directly rather than talking to you, when appropriate.
- Availability for extra time at appointments.
- Coverage when the dentist is away.
- Medical insurance accepted.
- Hospital affiliations.
- Availability of same-day appointments.

- Ease of referral to specialists.
- Willingness to partner with caregivers in addition to family members.
- Office location.

When we find a caring and helpful dentist, we become part of your marketing plan. We tell people. We share stories. We sing your praises. You can use social media, print advertising, and spend lots of money on your Web sites but, when you get down to figuring out where your referrals come from, you will most likely realize that there is no better advertising than the positive news that is spread by word of mouth.

You might want to know what we look for. Regardless of whether we bring a patient with a disability to your office, there are certain characteristics that are important when finding a dentist. We want to know:

- Are you compassionate, sensitive, and caring?
- Will you take the time to answer our questions?
- Are you considerate of our time and comfort?
- Do you demonstrate the professionalism and competency we expect?

## PAYING FOR SERVICES

You are probably wondering about whether seeing patients with ID/DDs will help your bottom line. Will we pay for services? Are they profitable patients?

Our children are eligible for private dental insurance as dependents of working parents. This important benefit can be maintained for our child as long as a parent is working and covered by an employer's health insurance program. This eligibility is maintained regardless of the age of the child.

Children with ID/DDs are as likely to come from families with the ability to pay easily for services as any other family.

Children without dental insurance who come from needy families, regardless of the presence of a disability, may be eligible for Medicaid.

As adults, some of our children will have access to their own private dental insurance through their employers or through their parents' employers. Others will have to rely on Medicaid or pay out of pocket.

Hopefully, through this textbook and new dental school curriculums, training for dentists on how to work with individuals with ID/DDs will reach more dental students. Historically, information on this special population has been included only in the curriculum for pediatric dentists. While attempts are under way to include training for adult dentists, many individuals with ID/DDs have continued to see their pediatric dentists into adulthood. Another reason for this is that the Medicaid reimbursement rates for dentists are so low that few adult dentists accept Medicaid.

Too often, however, adults with ID/DDs go without proper dental care because access and affordability are limited. Dental care may be an out-of-pocket expense. This is one of the reasons adults with disabilities receive monthly Social Security or Supplemental Security benefits—to pay for necessary expenses. I have also heard of parents or other family members who "treat" their child to a dental visit as a birthday present or for another special occasion.

I challenge you to be a WAIMDO, which means "welcome all in my dental office." This is a new slant to the NIMBY, which means "not in my backyard" and refers to people or groups who practice exclusionary zoning of one sort of another.

A WAIMDO is a dental office that accepts and celebrates differences. It recognizes that we are all differently abled. Hopefully you will be an excellent dentist, but you may struggle mightily at other things. And for those of us "abled," it is only temporary. If we live long enough, we all will experience disability.

Your practice will be one where trust and honesty are high and your commitment will reduce the anxiety of your patients. You will be committed to ensuring lifelong access to dental care either in your office or through referrals.

In return your dental office will be ensured a strong referral base based on the best kind of word-of-mouth advertising. You will enjoy a reputation of being thoughtful, patient, and kind. You will be talked about with only kind words at social gatherings. You will enjoy the highest level of social status—that of just a person.

When you eliminate the oral pain in someone with limited verbal skills, you will have developed new ways to use your skills and you will find that success is measured in different ways.

When you show that you care for a child with an ID/DD, you become a role model for your staff and for your other patients and their families. You might even give hope to a family at a time when they need it most. Families ache for those simple acts of acceptance. You will be given opportunities to impact lives in ways you never dreamed of.

Another true story: When my son finished his education and chose to begin his life 2 hours from our home, we had to find new medical and dental care. I began my search with finding a new internist. You already heard about Jon's dentist. He was not going to be replaced. I was going to do whatever it took for Jon to continue to see Dr. Perlman. It wasn't practical to change dentists, given Jon's complex and interesting medical situation (he was looking at another open heart surgery, a cardiac defibrillator, he used a CPAP machine, wore hearing aids, etc.). Changing doctors was daunting and scary. I wasn't up to meeting and interviewing doctors and their staff, but it had to be done. I started with getting recommendations from various people, both within and outside of the disability world. I made my first appointment with someone highly recommended. Competency was nonnegotiable. I was looking for those other qualities—kindness, compassion, and acceptance. Remember from the first story, my son was well-behaved and reserved. Still is. So I take him to the doctor's office and while waiting, I notice a commotion in the secretary's office area.

I see a woman I can tell has ID/DD having just finished her appointment, having a very difficult time. Instead of coming out into the waiting area, she sits down on the floor. She is being disruptive. I watch and here is what I see: Everyone in the waiting room continues to do what they were doing—reading magazines or continuing to stare into space. The staff in the area where the woman is having a hard time continue to go about their work. The staff person who was accompanying the woman reassures her and in 5 minutes is able to get her to stand up and leave the office.

I knew in that moment that this was an office where my son would be valued and welcomed. Based just on that interaction, and a very kind doctor, Jonathan found his new medical home. And I have been telling the story ever since.

# Epilogue

## International perspective
## Luc A.M. Marks, DDS, MSc, PhD

Treating the dental patient with a developmental disorder continues to be a big challenge in the twenty-first century. In this textbook, several topics are included to cover the range of problems that may arise while treating this group of patients. Most of the time the techniques described do not differ very much from treating the general population. However, when treating a patient with a developmental disorder, the dental practitioner needs to develop his or her skills to an extended level to deliver the appropriate services to the patient using the tools described in this textbook. Treating these patients in the general dental practice brings dentistry to a higher level. From an international perspective, treatment strategies are influenced by a variety of parameters.

In 2003, FDI (Fédération Dentaire Internationale), a global dental professional organization, published a policy statement supporting equal oral health care for special care patients. As a result, every dentist involved in this concept is supported by the general dental councilors from each individual country on the globe.

The Special Olympics Healthy Athletes Special Smiles initiative points out the existing oral health problems in the special care population since 1997 and can be seen as a mission that steers health care policy makers around the globe.

IADH (International Association for Disability and Oral Health) also created a global platform to discuss oral health care for special care patients, both clinically and scientifically, pointing out the problems that still exist.

*Treating the Dental Patient with a Developmental Disorder*, First Edition.
Edited by Karen A. Raposa and Steven P. Perlman.
© 2012 John Wiley & Sons, Inc. Published 2012 by John Wiley & Sons, Inc.

Dental schools can have a major influence in resolving some of these problems. Providing undergraduate students opportunities to treat this patient population can help create the change that is needed. When undergraduate students have very limited to no experience treating patients with developmental disorders, the result is most often a natural avoidance of the unknown during their entire professional career. Treatment of patients with developmental disorders during undergraduate training can make a major difference! Some schools around the globe have already incorporated the topic of the special care patient in their standard curriculum, including both theoretical and clinical training. In addition, it is becoming more common to see the creation of a special care platform within dental schools and a variety of departments bringing their knowledge together to treat special care patients. Historically, the pediatric dentist has been the dental professional who was trained to treat special care patients in most countries. However, additional knowledge related to periodontal problems, additional skills related to prosthetic rehabilitation, and expertise related to the medical problems of an adult and aging special care population can motivate dentists that are able, in collaboration with other health care professionals, to treat special care patients without any age limitations.

Similar to any new development in dentistry, it takes time to change the curriculum and methodologies that are currently being used in undergraduate training, especially when it comes to an ethical point of view of treating patients with developmental disorders. When reviewing the international perspective on treating the dental patient with a developmental disorder, ethical questions and considerations immediately come to mind. Cultures and habits differ all over the world. In the multicultural society we live in today, it seems almost intuitive to bring the best of all worlds into our own practice, which will allow our own ethical perspectives to be influenced. Since we have been influenced by the best practices in the world, we can no longer imagine dentistry being performed in a marketplace with someone holding a patient and someone else extracting a tooth.

It is critical that we assess the treatment we are currently delivering from an ethical point of view as well. We as practitioners should not be using different ethical principles when treating patients with developmental disorders as compared with our other patients. Techniques, methodologies, and principles are changing at galactic speeds in our world today. We should be striving to use some of the newest techniques, methodologies, and principles in our daily practices that make our patients feel as comfortable as possible during dental treatment.

As for patients with developmental disorders, the highest quality of dentist is needed, but it is important that dentists who are treating these patients not be punished financially. An investment in the prevention of oral disease in patients with developmental disorders from birth to elderly life is especially important.

Demographical changes are also influencing the population of patients with a developmental disorder. In the western world, the growth in the size of the aging population may place a burden on treatment of patients with developmental disorders, as a large portion of the efforts of dental practitioners may be focused on aging patients. However, one might argue that this shift may result in more practitioners feeling comfortable with treating special care patients. It should be noted that developing countries with a young population appear to have increased their efforts toward treating special care patients.

Now is the time to change our attitudes and treatment perspective and to create a platform for the need for more dental practitioners who are skilled in caring for patients with developmental disorders, since their needs will increase drastically throughout the years. All authors in this book have tried to provide a contribution and perspective related to this existing need.

## REFERENCES

FDI World Dental Federation (Fédération Dentaire Internationale), www.FDIworldental.org.

International Association for Disability and Oral Health, www.iadh.org.

Special Olympics, www.specialolympics.com.

# Index

*Treating the Dental Patient with a Developmental Disorder*, First Edition.
Edited by Karen A. Raposa and Steven P. Perlman.
© 2012 John Wiley & Sons, Inc. Published 2012 by John Wiley & Sons, Inc.

Printed and bound by CPI Group (UK) Ltd, Croydon, CR0 4YY

16/04/2025

14658468-0001

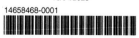